Medical school is a whirlwind experience, a crash course in science and practice, but also in healing and humanity. . . . The true heroism I see day to day is in the enormous patience, diligence, and quiet care given by physicians to patients.

There must be, however, room for criticism. Due to the enormous power of physicians over people, not only through medicine, but through their language, actions, and attitudes, those in the medical field cannot be afraid to critically examine the images we use day to day. . . . Rather than maintaining a "don't ask, don't tell" policy regarding self-criticism, it's time to bite the bullet.

And I, the Private Benjamin of the medical world, will continue to plod through my practice drills, waiting for the time when my number is called. When that time comes, I can only hope to be a lover and not a fighter. . . .

HER OWN MEDICINE:

A Woman's Journey
from Student to Doctor

Sayantani DasGupta, M.D., M.P.H.

FAWCETT GOLD MEDAL • NEW YORK

A Fawcett Gold Medal Book
Published by The Ballantine Publishing Group
Copyright © 1999 by Sayantani DasGupta

Grateful acknowledgment is made to the following for permission to reprint previously published material:

American Medical Student Association: "A Bitter Bullet" by Sayantani DasGupta. First published in *The New Physician*, November 1996, © 1996 American Medical Student Association. Reprinted by permission of the American Medical Student Association.

Annals of Behavioral Science and Medical Education: "Models, Mentors and Motherhood: Bringing Up Future Female Physicians" by Sayantani DasGupta. This article (copyright 1996 by the Association for the Behavioral Sciences and Medical Education) is being reprinted with the permission of ABSAME as it appeared in the *Annals of Behavioral Science and Medical Education* (Spring 1996, Volume 3 Issue 1, pages 3–5).

Contemporary Pediatrics: "Song of the Dying Ova" from *Contemporary Pediatrics* resident supplement, © 1995 Medical Economics Company. Used with permission.

www.randomhouse.com/BB/

Library of Congress Catalog Card Number: 99-90465

ISBN 0-449-00309-4

Printed in Canada

First Edition: October 1999

10 9 8 7 6 5 4 3 2

For beloved Ma and Baba.

Contents

Introduction

___

The scene opens on a desert battle. From the sky beats down not only an unmerciful sun but torrents of intermittent shelling. A group of soldiers are huddling together in a shallow trench. Although they occasionally arise to fire on an unseen enemy, they primarily stay within their makeshift home, holding each other for comfort. Suddenly, the air is filled with a noxious, frightening odor. Nerve gas? Chemical warfare? No, of course not. A female soldier straightens her stethoscope and smooths the lapel of her white coat. The smell makes her eyes water with exhaustion and emotion. It's formaldehyde.

Medicine, like the military, is a historically male-dominated sphere. It was not until the mid-1970s that medical schools began to see an increasing number of women students, and not until very recently that women physicians entered the ranks of senior faculty and deans at medical schools. Despite growing numbers, however, it is clear that both medicine and the military have often reacted with hostility to their female soldiers.

Since the sexual harassment scandal hit the military, it seems that every time I turn on the television, there are new reports of violence, harassment, and hazing in the armed forces. From women being forced to "run the gauntlet" at the Tailhook Convention, to the Citadel driving away female student after female student, to the highly publicized cases of sexual misconduct of the Aberdeen Proving Grounds, it is clear that while official policies may have changed, the military old boys' club still does not respond well to women in their midst. As Carol Burke, a former professor from the U.S. Naval Academy observes, "In civilian life, there has clearly been a re-examination of gender roles and of what masculinity is . . . [but] there is a nostalgia in the military for an institution you could count on to confer manhood to its members."[1] Like the military, medicine, too, is an institution that has not caught up with modern gender politics.

I in no way mean to trivialize the plight of female soldiers. The overt violence faced by many military women is not often shared by their sisters in medicine. Despite its more covert nature, however, medical sexism is alive and well in many hospitals and teaching institutions. The well-publicized 1991 resignation of neurosurgeon Dr. Frances K. Conley from Stanford University and her subsequent charges of pervasive sexism in medicine is but one example. In a 1992 *JAMA* article, Dr. Conley writes, "The hierarchy of 'good old boys' . . . is dedicated to preservation of its upper echelon in its own image . . . lady members are rarely allowed to forget that they are there by invitation, are expected to demonstrate eternal gratitude, and always to obey the rules."[2] Charges of a "glass ceiling," "club" exclusion, an atmosphere of subtle

[1] Christine A. Rowett, "Bringing the Military to Attention," *The Gazette,* 26, no. 9 (7 April 1997):1, 9.
[2] Frances K. Conley, " . . . And, Ladies of the Club," *JAMA,* 267, no. 5 (5 February 1992):740–41.

sexism, and medical "microinequities" have been made by numerous women physicians.[3] Whether it is being passed up for a deserved promotion, being forced to listen to demeaning jokes about women, or having one's authority undermined by colleagues, women physicians in the 1990s have to work within an oftentimes unfriendly environment.

But what about the "changing face of medicine"? Wasn't all of that Old Boys stuff supposed to be a thing of the past? That was what I was led to believe when I was applying for medical school in the early 1990s. Perhaps as a reaction to the powerful influence of the managed-care revolution, medical schools in the early 1990s were portraying themselves as female-friendly institutions interested in holistic care, psychosocial issues, and well-rounded students. My own decision to apply to medical school was heavily influenced by these sentiments. I became convinced that the institution of medicine was ripe for change, and that I would be a welcome representative of the "new wave." I believed the media image, that medical schools were filled to the brim with unusual students such as professional National Geographic photographers, Peace Corps volunteers who had raised llamas in Peru, and adventurers who had scaled Mount Everest. I was thrilled at the exciting prospect of

[3] Janet Bickel, "Leveling the Playing Field: A National Perspective on Sexism and Professional Development in Medicine," in *Women in Medical Education*, Delese Wear, ed., (Albany, N.Y.: State University of New York Press, 1996): 11–20; Frances K. Conley, "Toward a More Perfect World—Eliminating Sexual Discrimination in Academic Medicine," *The New England Journal of Medicine*, (4 February 1993): 351–52; Randi Henderson, "Women in the Promised Land," *Hopkins Medical News* (winter 1994): 38–45.

working in such a dynamic and open environment. I was in for a rude awakening.

Johns Hopkins Medical School has a historical debt to women. Although the hospital began operations in 1887, it did not possess the funds to assemble the faculty and finish constructing the medical school. The medical school, which opened in 1893, was funded by four wealthy Baltimore women, who raised and donated a total of $500,000 on the stipulation that "women be admitted to the School on the same terms as men."[4] These women further stipulated that the bequest be published annually in the School of Medicine Catalog (where it can still be seen today), that a women's advisory committee be maintained, and that a pre-medical course of study be required for admission of all medical students.[5] Thus, Johns Hopkins has not only admitted women students since its inception, but its high standard of medical education was set by a group of women.

The problem, thus, can hardly be considered a historic lack of inclusion. Nor can it be inclusion by numbers, since my medical school class entering in 1993 was approximately 45 percent women, while the class below me was about 51 percent female students. The problem is more imperceptible. It involves the subtle and not so subtle culture of medicine that seeps into a woman's skin only after she is well entrenched in the field. As Janet Bickel from the Association of American Medical Col-

[4] E. B. Thomas, "How Women Medical Students First Came to Johns Hopkins: A Chronicle," Caroline Bedell Thomas Papers, Sophia Smith Collection, Smith College, Northampton, Mass., 1975 as referred to in Joseph B. Shrager, "Three Women at Johns Hopkins: Private Perspectives on Medical Coeducation in the 1890s," *Annals of Internal Medicine* 115, no. 7 (October 1991): 56–69.
[5] Shrager, "Three Women at Johns Hopkins," 564–69.

leges writes, "many women face lonely decisions about how to deal with a broad range of 'microinequities'—from deliberate exploitation to unconscious slights ... while some microinequities may look as harmless as a drop of water, as a persistent drip, they can wear a woman down, interfere with her work, and exact costly tolls on self-confidence and relationships."[6]

My experience at Johns Hopkins Medical School, an institution famed for its medical leadership as well as its historic inclusion of women, confirms Bickel's sentiments. Indeed, when I arrived at Hopkins in 1993, bright-eyed and bushy-tailed about my new chosen profession, I was hardly prepared for my unfamiliar new environment. I came from a fairly liberal New England college, Brown University, having studied as much anthropology and literary criticism as biology. My time at Brown was spent with various activist groups, but I soon grew disenchanted, wondering what good protesting about inequality was if one did not do anything practical about it. I came to think of medicine as a concrete way to effect social change, and impact the lives of women and children, minority communities, and the economically disadvantaged.

I came to medical school having had no medical role models, no physicians in my close family or circle of friends. My image of the medical profession was shaped by childhood episodes of *M*A*S*H* and *St. Elsewhere*. I thought of physicians as idealistic movers and shakers, their worst quality being that they were sometimes womanizers, if of the liberal, Alan Alda–variety. As a teenager, I was hooked on a short-lived TV show about a

[6] Janet Bickel, "Leveling the Playing Field," 11–20.

holistic women's health center. Although the program
was canceled shortly after it first aired, it was enough to
whet my appetite. It showed me a vision not only of female physicianhood, but of a type of medicine that fit my
politics, my social goals. I did not know what flaming
hoops I would have to jump through to come close to
achieving that fantasy. I did not know not to believe
everything I saw on TV.

"In order to write this book I had to go to medical
school,"[7] writes Perri Klass in *A Not Entirely Benign
Procedure*, a 1987 book of essays about a woman's experiences at Harvard Medical School. Ten years later, I
have experienced some of the same pressures Klass described, as well as a host of new adventures determined
by the managed-care revolution, the changed economy,
and AIDS. My experiences also differ from Dr. Klass's in
that I am an Indian American woman, a dark-skinned
daughter of foreign immigrants. As such, my childhood
was intermittently plagued with schoolmate "anthropolo-
gists" fascinated by my skin, my hair, my funny name. I
was asked, on more than one occasion, whether my "tan"
came off, whether I ate snakes, or slept in a teepee, and
why I wouldn't just "go back where I came from." I became supersensitized to the contradictions of cultures,
the explosions that often take place when different
worlds collide. I still cringe when my medical colleagues,
who are all accustomed to pronouncing long Latin-
derived microbiologic and pharmacological names,
struggle over mine. It isn't easy to have your performance remembered by your attending physicians when

---

[7] Perri Klass, *A Not Entirely Benign Procedure,* (New York: Signet,
1987).

they can't even remember your name. This collection of essays documents the journey of the medical student immigrant through her new homeland: the diverse, complex, and sometimes oppressive world of medicine.

While I am the daughter of immigrants, I am also the daughter of a feminist mother, who has for all my life been involved in women's movements both within and without our Indian American community. In fact, one of my earliest memories is marching in a "Take Back the Night" rally hand-in-hand with my mother. I was inculcated into the culture of activism at a tender age, and read as much Gloria Steinem as Beatrix Potter. I am what is now fashionably called a "second generation feminist," and so my vision is finely calibrated to sense gender inequity.

Her Own Medicine was born out of necessity. Like Perri Klass, I, too, had to go to medical school to write this book; in addition, I had to write this book to survive medical school. Putting pen to paper, or in my case, fingers to keyboard, has always been a way for me to make sense of the world around me. While it's not something I might advertise to my administration, I only got through some of the tougher times at medical school by imagining myself as an anthropologist doing field work. I navigated the day-to-day rigors of the hospital by taking mental field notes on the culture and rituals of the medical "natives." I imagined myself in a pith hat and khaki safari jacket, the Jane Goodall to their medical monkey antics.

The first, and the perhaps most blatant, aspect of medical culture that struck me upon entering medical school was its similarity to the military. "If you look at the transition period in most branches of service from civilian life and civilian identity to military life and military identity," says Carol Burke, "you see a very conscious effort on the part of military institutions to erase an old individuality and substitute a corporate one."[8] Similarly, medical education is designed to "transform an ordinary person into a doctor."[9] From the first day, medical school, too, marks a transition from "civilian life" to "physician life," a change from individual to collective, medical identity.

In the military, as Burke says, "you take away the clothes, you shave the hair, you deprive them of sleep, you yell and scream at them."[10] While there isn't any ritualistic shaving, medical school does determine our schedules, our language, and our white-coated uniform. Like the military, too, medical training is strictly hierarchical, with med-student privates, intern lieutenants, resident sergeants, and fellow captains. Young faculty members are, perhaps, the majors, while the old faculty are definitely the generals. The first two years of medical school, when my platoon of 120 students was shepherded from basic science classroom to basic science classroom and taught the fundamentals of biochemistry, anatomy, physiology, pharmacology, and pathology, were like boot camp. They were rigorous, but obviously only a prelude to actual battle.

The last two years of medical school, students are thrown into hospital frontline duty and go through "rotations" in the various medical disciplines including

[8] Rowett, "Bringing the Military."
[9] Debra Roter and Judith Hall, *Doctors Talking with Patients, Patients Talking with Doctors: Improving Communication in Medical Visits* (Westport, CT: Auburn House, 1992).
[10] Rowett, "Bringing the Military."

surgery, internal medicine, obstetrics and gynecology (OB/Gyn), pediatrics, psychiatry, neurology, ophthalmology, and emergency medicine. The wards are both challenging and invigorating. These are the times a student gets to interact with and impact the lives of patients. Unfortunately, more time is often spent with physician teachers than patients. Physicians teach students the day-to-day practicalities of medicine, as well as reinforce their theoretical background. However, the means by which students learn are often more than Socratic; "pimping" is the term used to describe the often obtuse, often obscure, rapid-fire questions students are posed by their senior physicians. Clinical rotations require a student to always be "on"—ready to draw correct answers from the dark recesses of one's memory at the slightest provocation. Thus, rotations become like tours of duty, each one a new opportunity to impress or disappoint a hierarchical team of doctors.

When on the wards in the hospital, one does not break rank, but takes direct orders from interns, who in turn answer to senior residents, who in turn report to the attending physician faculty members. I remember during one of my early rotations, I could not find any intern, and so had my medical orders (including IV-fluid rates, medicines, and nursing specifics) on a patient overlooked and co-signed by the senior resident. The resident did not seem to think anything of it, but my intern screamed her head off at me. I learned not to break the rules of hierarchy again.

It is not just students who must follow these rigid rules, either. Rank-and-file surgical and medical residents call their supervisory attending physicians "Sir" (although I have never heard a female attending being

called "Ma'am"). One surgical resident I know named
Jack is consistently called "Dan" by the head of his department. Jack now answers to "Dan," since, as he ex-
plains, you just don't correct your chief, even if he calls
you by the wrong name.

More than these spectacles of hierarchy and tradition,
however, medicine's similarity to the military is seen in
its use of language. In fact, physicians and physicians-in-
training propagate and celebrate this likeness through
militarylike metaphors. One of the favorites among my
medical school classmates was "gunner." A Webster's
definition of the word might look something like this:
gunner *(noun)*—a cutthroat competitive student; a nerd;
among the medical elite, a term of begrudging, jealous
admiration; *(verb)*—to compete; to study; as in the sentence, "You gotta **gun** away on that pharm exam, attack
it with all your guns blazin'!" Occasionally, when said
with a drawl, the term can stand on its own, a testament
to the speaker's and listener's common participation in
the same war. Then, the word is a passing call-to-arms,
"Gun-neerrr!!!"

Not only students, but physicians at all levels of
training participate in this festival of military metaphors.
Doctors are "in the trenches" and "on the front line," radiation "blasts" through cancer, while large doses of antibiotics "bomb" infections. A recent talk I attended on
stereotachtic, or ultrasound-guided, needle breast biop-
sies made the metaphor glaringly obvious by inter-
spersing tactical military maps among the slides of the
procedure itself. "Like a stealth missile, the needle can
zoom directly in on its target," the speaker gloated, flip-
ping through military satellite pictures of targeted areas
juxtaposed with pictures of women's breasts. "We can

zap the tumor, just like that, and then move on to obliterate the cancer altogether." Indeed, technology used in the Gulf War to create images of Baghdad is now being used to screen breast cancer in a program called "Missiles to Mammograms."

Ultimately, the end result of medicine's similarity to the military is the way it molds its soldiers. "What [military training] does is break down the individual and make him a follower," says Burke. "That's a somewhat risky process when waging wars demands both followers and leaders."[11] The same can be said of medical training. Indeed, the "pre-med syndrome" has already been described by scholars of medical education as one with the signs and symptoms of "aggressive competitiveness, self-interested pursuit of grades, narrow-minded overspecialization, high anxiety, and more than occasional incidents of academic dishonesty."[12] The rigorous process of medical training only takes these traits and amplifies them, to deleterious ends for both practitioners and patients. Indeed, "the [medical] educational experience is structured to militate against the development of humanistic doctor-patient relationships ... [physicians-in-training] are systematically dehumanized, which only fosters the deterioration of the doctor-patient relationship rather than allowing it to develop as something positive."[13]

Like the military, women are allowed to join the ranks

[11] Ibid.

[12] R. Fox, *Essays in Medical Sociology: Journeys Into the Field* (New Brunswick, N.J.: Transaction Books, 1989), as referred in Roter and Hall, "Doctors Talking."

[13] T. Mizrahi, *Getting Rid of Patients: Contradictions in the Socialization of Physicians* (New Brunswick, N.J.: Rutgers University Press, 1986), as referred in Roter and Hall.

of the medical elite. So, too, have some women risen up through the ranks to positions of power. However, the underlying masculine culture of medicine has not much changed, except in limited circumstances and in certain fields such as pediatrics and to some extent OB/Gyn. Sexist jokes, masculine rituals, and rigid rules create an invisible but very formidable fortress around those women who breach the barricades of medical training. To protect themselves, many women who have "made it" in the medical hierarchy have had to build "suits of armor" around themselves.[14] Unfortunately, these very women sometimes continue to propagate the old-boys culture, subjecting younger women to the same rigors they themselves suffered.

So how does a female medical private survive this on-slaught of med-school mortar? Again, we perhaps need look no further than our sisters in uniform to understand survival strategies. Indeed, alongside cases of male offi-cers harassing female recruits have been an increas-ing number of recent court-martials involving female military officers accused of having extramarital affairs—which is considered, in military terms, "conduct unbe-coming an officer and *a gentleman*." As a medical private myself, I know that the most natural way to survive in war is to take comfort from those around you. Human relationships, both romantic and platonic, are the key to surviving on at least the medical battlefront.

Other medical students are, of course, the first line of defense. Each incoming class, like a platoon or squad-ron, experiences medical initiation on the same timeline.

[14] Marjorie S. Sirridge, "Special Armor," *Women in Medical Education*, Delese Wear, ed., (Albany, N.Y.: State University of New York, 1996), 159–64.

They study together, play together, work in the hospital together, cram together, and more often than not, romance together. Not only fellow medical privates are sources of potential support, however. Physician mentors, nurses, health-care ancillary personnel, patients, and patients' families provide anchoring and perspective— granting human relationships in an oftentimes war-torn environment.

The problem, then, for young women physicians is the dearth of healthy, supportive human relationships that accept us for who we are and encourage us to grow into who we can become. I was lucky enough to find a supportive male partner, a handful of wonderful female friends, and some physicians, nurses, and patients who have made my journey easier. These relationships were, however, the exception. In the militaristic medical culture of Hopkins, it was difficult for me to find role models, or even colleagues, who marched to my kinder, gentler drummer. Indeed, beyond the sheer intellectual and physical rigor, the emotional drain of this type of solitary warfare was so great that I required an entire year of R and R before I could return to the front. In between my third and fourth years of medical school, I escaped to do a masters of public health (MPH) at the Johns Hopkins School of Hygiene and Public Health, an environment as supportive as medical school was isolating, as invigorating as medical school was demoralizing.

Being away from the battlefront, however, only made me more vulnerable. It made me see the problems more clearly, and, like the soldier who suddenly wonders what all the violence is for, it made me question more fundamentally the nature of medical training. I realized that medical school had been four years "in the trenches," and that most of the time, I had felt like I was running, head down, through a battlefield with mortar blasts exploded all around me. As I wrote this book, more clearly articulating problems in medical education even to myself, I found myself growing into more and more of a pacifist. Like some incongruous soldier-turned-antiwar protester, I imagined myself wearing love beads over fatigues, braids under a helmet, and making a peace sign with two fingers instead of holding a gun. With each essay, I learned; with each word, I grew.

The essays of this collection are categorized in quite literally a sequential order, as witness to my experiences as I undertook them. They fall under four basic headings: basic science years and clinical experiences are sandwiched between a brief introductory section about medicine and militarism in general, and a longer last section focusing on gender issues in medicine. The headings themselves are as follows: *Of Gunners, Marines, and Mortar*—the sole essay in this section, "A Bitter Bullet: Medicine as Militarism," sets the tone for the rest of this book by making clear the analogies between medicine and militarism; *Boot Camp: The Preclinical Years*—these pieces describe two very different experiences I had during the first two years of medical school: beginning a relationship with my future husband, and losing a medical school friend to cancer; *In the Trenches: The Clinical Years*—the essays in this section describe the different clinical rotations of the third and fourth years of medical school, including emergency medicine, pediatrics, OB/Gyn, internal medicine, surgery, psychiatry, a foreign rotation, the harrowing process of choosing a residency, and finally, the frightening transition from medical school to internship. The last section, *The Gender Wars,* summarizes some gender-related issues in medical training, including the relationships between female medical students and the need for female physician mentors. These essays offer a solution to the problems of gender inequity in medicine: changing the culture of medicine itself to support women physicians; creating a world where we can practice our own medicine.

The essays in this volume span a wide range of topics, including clinical rotations, romance in the hospital, AIDS, mentoring, and media portrayals of medical professionals. This book is both a set of personal reflections and a glimpse into the world of medical training in the 1990s. It critiques the medical establishment's treatment of its female recruits toward the purpose of making medical culture more woman-friendly. Only by demystifying the age-old traditions of medical training can a new environment be created, which is both more supportive of physicians and healthier for patients. *Her Own Medicine* aims at being part of that solution. It is meant to amuse and provoke, illustrate problems and suggest solutions. Ultimately, it is a compilation of stories from the front lines; not of a battle, but of a dynamic and rich field defined by the very humanity of both its patients and its practitioners.

Of Gunners,
Marines, and
Mortar

A Bitter Bullet:
Medicine as Militarism

I've always loved the movie *Private Benjamin*. While I am hardly a proponent of militarism, there's something about that film with which I have always been able to identify. I used to think it was the feminist message about a woman who finds her voice and makes it, as it were, in "this man's army." Little did I know, however, that I would have something in common with Goldie Hawn's long-ago character. It's not that I've given up my pacifist principles and joined the U.S. military. Yet, my training in one of this country's most famous medical schools harkens back to Goldie's Private Benjamin.

During my experiences in the hospital wards, I became more and more convinced of the insidious similarities between medicine and the military. Indeed, these similarities are actually encouraged in day-to-day medical life. In honor of Johns Hopkins Hospital's first chairman of medicine, particularly stalwart Hopkins medical residents are still called "Osler Marines."

While my days and nights on the wards can hardly be compared to Bosnia, I've seen my fair share of medical mortar exploding in the hospital hallways. And I, the naive medical private, have more than once, like Benjamin, wondered what exactly I've gotten myself into.

We're in the Army Now

Medical initiates are quite similar to military "grunts" who sweat through rigorous weeks of boot camp. As boot camp breaks down civilians to create good soldiers, so, too, does medical training try to mold individuals into a common idea of a good physician. In the case of medical school, boot camp is the first two years of classroom learning, during which students are herded from class to class, with little autonomy or room for creativity, and inundated with endless facts to memorize. If the first two years of medical training are boot camp, the last two, during which students are thrown onto the hospital wards, are definitely frontline duty.

Private Benjamin, upon receiving her army greens, responded with the plaintive cry, "Do these come in another color?" In medicine, the white coat is our uniform. Like squadrons of soldiers, we white-coated troops march about the medical hallways, led by our senior resident sergeants and attending physician generals. The uniform is not merely a circumstance, but a symbol of belonging to the institution of medicine. Indeed, before beginning our clinical years, the medical students at my school attended a "white coat ceremony" in which we were presented with our garb in a ritual of medical glory. "Never forget, you are entering an honored and ancient profession," numerous speakers told us. "It is you who will welcome new life into this world, and it will be your face that some poor soul sees before drawing his or her dying breath."

The keynote speaker at this event regaled us with stories from the front. "I had to miss my son's fifth birthday party because of an emergency pediatric surgery," he explained, "but when I got home, I told my disappointed son, 'I didn't have time to get you a toy, but this year, for your birthday present, I saved another child's life.' " To the stunned audience's reaction, the speaker added, "and my son thanked me." I wasn't sure if I was supposed to cry, salute, or break into an impromptu chorus of "Over There."

In the Trenches

The language of militarism is much used in medical practice. In keeping with the germ theory, the enemy of choice is usually disease. However, too often, the enemy is the patient. Indeed, in the much-beleaguered life of the medical intern, incoming patients are "hits" to be avoided. This mentality, while a coping mechanism for a stressful job, too often translates into physician behavior.

"Don't take any crap from that sickler," I was told regarding a patient with sickle cell anemia, "she's a frequent flyer here, and a drug seeker." Later, I would hear that physician barking at the woman when she refused to have a rectal examination. "You have no right to refuse this exam. It's part of your care," the doctor bellowed. "You can't pick and choose what you want in the hospital, you know. You walk in our door, you give up that right." Clearly, that pillar of the medical community had never heard of the Bill of Rights. Or, at least, thought that it didn't apply in our hospital.

During another late evening, I found myself interviewing the family of Mrs. A., an elderly lady suspected of having pancreatic cancer. Mrs. A.'s daughters, distressed by her condition as well as her deteriorating mental status, weren't exactly cogent history givers. However, they were warm, charming, and ultimately gave me the appropriate information. In the middle of my interview, the red-eyed intern rushed in. "Sorry, but I have to interrupt," he said, seating himself in the chair one of Mrs. A.'s daughters had been occupying. "Let's start from the beginning, OK? And when I'm done, Dr . . . ahhh," he looked at me. "What's your name again?" I answered. "Right. Well, afterward, she can ask you anything she likes."

"Well," began the particularly long-winded one, while the other, now chairless, shifted uncomfortably around, "we had just gone to Florida. To Walt Disney World, you know? Have you ever been there?"

As the interview dragged interminably on, the intern grew exasperated. "Look, let's try and at least stick to the point. I have a lot of patients waiting for me in the emergency room, and I don't have all night for this. Do you think you can manage to stay focused for five minutes?" I felt ashamed, and couldn't meet the eyes of the two middle-aged ladies, each old enough to be my, and the intern's, mother. My previous jovial conversation with them made me want to be their ally. But I was in a white coat, and that made the rude intern my comrade, and them the enemy.

A Children's Crusade

The patient as the enemy is a disheartening idea in any situation. However, when the enemy on the other side of the medical front line is a child, it is even more disturbing. During my pediatrics rotation, I saw more than one "difficult child" ignored by medical and nursing staff, while pleasant children, who were usually the ones with significant family and social support anyway, got a disproportionate amount of friendly attention.

One such "difficult child" was an eight-year-old girl admitted for vaginal pain and a vulvar rash. While the child was not difficult in behavior, she was perhaps an "unsavory" pediatric patient, due to her impoverished socioeconomic status, and the sexual nature of her illness. On first glance, the girl was older than her years, yet her facial expression made her look even younger than eight. She looked stoically at the ceiling, clutching a teddy bear while our team each examined her vagina in turn. Her mother walked distractedly about the room, wringing her hands. "How will I tell her father?" she kept asking. "He'll go crazy. Couldn't it be something else?" But the lesions were unmistakable.

"Your daughter has genital herpes," the attending physician said bluntly to the mother. "I suggest you keep a closer eye on her." In the hallway, his discussion was equally blunt. "I'm discharging this patient now. Why the hell was she admitted anyway? Herpes can be treated as an outpatient." When I asked, weakly, whether we should consider the safety of the young girl's home environment, the doctor cut me off. "She's a Tanner three, at least," he said, and walked away, implying that the girl was high on the Tanner scale of pubertal development, and thus her sexual activity must have been consensual.

Before the team was done rounding, the girl was gone. Guilt-ridden and unable to sleep well that night, I mentioned the incident to another attending physician the next day, who immediately notified the girl's private doctor. However, the fact remains that a probable victim of sexual abuse was shooed off the ward back to her likely environment of abuse.

The Big General in the Sky

In the environment where any new patient is an unwanted crash of mortar fire, the loss of a patient is a physician victory. Unfortunately, many times, this loss of a patient from the service is to death. "At least I don't have to check her labs anymore," an intern once commented upon the death of her patient.

Mrs. A., the woman with the verbose children, also eventually died, to which my intern replied, "Well, I'm not shedding any tears." He was, perhaps, happy that he did not have to hear about Walt Disney World anymore.

Physicians are not, however, always heartless. A senior resident once told me, "Mr. B. isn't on our service anymore." To my naive and confused questions as to where exactly the patient had gone, the resident explained, "He's on a better service. God's."

Magic Bullets

Medical school is a whirlwind experience, a crash course in science and practice, but also in healing and humanity. It is, as well, a lesson of how to survive in a somewhat hostile environment. Indeed, the high tensions of medicine often make the source of hospital hallway mortar the "friendly fire" from bitter fellow physicians. Yet, despite numerous less-than-ideal medical situations

I have observed, I also have seen many heroic actions on the part of my physician mentors. The problem is, unlike on medical dramas, the true heroism I see day to day is in the enormous patience, diligence, and quiet care given by physicians to patients.

There must be, however, room for criticism. Due to the enormous power of physicians over people, not only through medicine, but through their language, actions, and attitudes, those in the medical field cannot be afraid to critically examine the images we use day to day. In the modern-day world of medicine, where health care changes are undercutting the idea of "physician as God," and increasing numbers of women are toppling traditional male leadership, we must question the use of military metaphors in medical care. There is no magic bullet to solving the "patient as enemy"/"physician as marine" opposition beyond our own awareness that these seemingly powerless ideas significantly influence our behavior and attitudes. Rather than maintaining a "don't ask, don't tell" policy regarding self-criticism, it's time to bite the bullet.

And I, the Private Benjamin of the medical world, will continue to plod through my practice drills, waiting for the time when my number is called. When that time comes, I can only hope to be a lover, and not a fighter.

Boot Camp:
The Preclinical
Years

Love in the
Time of Formaldehyde

Even bad movies about life in medical school have their own peculiar formulas. Romance is an integral component of good medical education and even the worst movies do their best to portray it. Take Julia Roberts and Kevin Bacon in *Flatliners*; OK, the movie was ridiculous (what first year medical student is capable of performing any sort of surgery, let alone surgical adventures in the netherworld?), but the romance portrayed was critical. Even nerds, it is clear, deserve love.

The first year of medical school, which brings together 100 to 150 overachieving young people, can perhaps be likened to a super-intellectual dating service. Since few medical students actually have the looks of a Julia Roberts or Kevin Bacon, and pre-med life is a bit more hectic than Hollywood, medical school is often the first time for future doctors to seek romance. At my school, orientation week was like a hormonally charged shopping spree, with men and women checking out the merchandise under the guise of meeting their colleagues to be. "We always get at least five or six marriages within each medical school class," a dean commented during orientation, "and at least half of you will find your future husbands and wives while you are in medical school."

Our overcrowded living arrangements—a medical school dorm that housed about 60 percent of our first-year class—did nothing to dilute the pheromone frenzy. Everyone was eager to show how laid-back, noncompetitive and non-nerdy they were, so the first few weeks of medical school were like a fraternity beer bash. Premeds who had been confined to the world of beakers and Bunsen burners in college were suddenly free to frolic, and romances bloomed and faded willy-nilly in the dorm.

The rules of romance among the medical elite are unique. For instance, although my classmates and I were to be the future of U.S. health care, our collective romantic behavior more closely resembled the behavior of kindergartners. Gossip was the rule of the day, so that any stray look, any token of affection, and any night spent in a room that was not one's own was immediately considered communal information. The romantic antics of my classmates ranged from the ridiculous to the, well, utterly ridiculous. The worst story I ever heard involved an alleged stalking. Contrary to what one might believe, however, it was a woman who stalked a male classmate, calling him incessantly, leaving him notes, and even showing up at his house until he found it necessary to actually call the police. While I can't vouch for the truth of this little piece of gossip, it makes me think that HMOs aren't the only reason we have to worry about the future of health care.

After the frenzied couplings and uncouplings of the first year, the next burst of romantic escapades in my medical school class occurred during our third year, when we were released from the basic science classroom and set loose on the hospital wards. As any med school movie, hospital TV drama, or soap opera worth its salt will tell you, a hospital is fertile ground for romance. Each nine-week rotation, when medical students are paired with teams from various medical specialties, is also an opportunity to meet and mate. Although medical students are strongly discouraged from dating their supervisory interns and residents, rotations are often the time when medical students become friendly with future romantic interests. Not only do medical students find romance with residents, but with nurses, dietitians, rehabilitation specialists, and other ancillary staff in the hospital. As much as the thought might churn the stomach, the rumor is that the tiny cubicle-like call rooms in the hospital are not always used for just sleeping.

Personally, I did not even make it past the first year's coupling melee. Cupid's arrow caught me during that fateful class of all medical school classes, Gross Anatomy. The odd thing is, my cupid was a cadaver.

The first day of Anatomy lab, when we nervously entered that den of formaldehyde that was to be our home for the next three months, one student actually fainted. I won't say that I wasn't tempted to do the same. Nothing prepares you for the experience of entering an eerily cold and silent room lit by flickering fluorescent overheads, filled with bodybags. Once inside the room, four students to a body-laden table, I could not help but feel that we had stepped into our own bad med school movie. I glanced surreptitiously around for a hidden camera.

My strongest memories of Gross Anatomy are all visceral. I remember the overly bright lights, the clammy, hard-to-cut skin of the cadavers, the floors slippery from formaldehyde, tissue, and unidentifiable body fluids. My strongest memory of all, however, is the smell. The smell of formaldehyde, for those who have never experienced

it, is an indescribably pungent, revolting, and invasive
stench. Through layers of scrubs, jackets, and plastic
aprons, the smell seeped into my underclothes and skin.
Despite slathering gobs of Vaseline on my hands (an
age-old med student odor-barrier trick) before donning
two pairs of gloves, my hands reeked even after multiple
washings. The smell was in my bedroom, hair, and pores.
I threw away stained and stinking lab coats, covered my
hair with bandannas, and designated certain scrubs,
socks, and bras for Anatomy use only, washing them over
and over with industrial-strength detergent.

Cadaver dissection is perhaps the prototypic medical school experience. Such intimate interaction with a
human body is both awe-inspiring and desensitizing.
Dissection is, however, more than the mere experience
of removing flesh, uncovering organ systems, and tracing
the complicated twists and turns of blood vessels. It is a
cultural experience all its own, an initiation into the
myths and realities of medicine. Dissection removes
much of the mystery around death, and conveys upon
young people a feeling of power over the human body. It
is ironic that it was during this very raw experience, this
exploration into both the gross and the anatomic, that I
was to begin a relationship with my future husband.

It was a romance straight out of an episode of the *Twilight Zone*. He was working at a table close to mine, and
one evening, we were the only people in the lab, both
preparing for presentations. The overhead lights flick-
ered eerily and the smell of formaldehyde hung nause-
atingly in the air. I wouldn't have been surprised if
Frankenstein had risen up from one of the tables. Then,
something happened. He looked at me, I looked at him,
and someone smiled. In that cloyingly creepy environ-

ment, we couldn't help but be grateful we were young and healthy and alive. We started to laugh at ourselves, two relatively happy-go-lucky people slaving away in the middle of the night in the anatomy lab. I had been momentarily desensitized to how surreal the scene actually was, and being able to share the experience put it in perspective. We put some Motown on the disgusting, formaldehyded radio in the room, and boogied while dissecting. Unbeknownst to our nosy classmates, our friendship soon progressed to a laughter-filled romance. We memorized Anatomy by setting medical lyrics to our favorite danceable songs. While other couples might discuss body parts in a more suggestive fashion, all of our early romantic dialogues involved gross anatomy.

Wrapping his arm around my neck, my boyfriend would murmur huskily, "Baby, you're the aorta and I'm your recurrent laryngeal nerve,"—describing the anatomic position of those two parts of the human body.

Not to be outdone, I would rumble anatomic lyrics to Sade's "Smooth Operator" in my best smoky voice.

"Smooth Obturator ... Smooth Obturator ..." I would sing.

I'm sure Sade never imagined her sexy hit would be used to describe a thigh muscle. The clincher was the verse about the pelvic nerve innervating the male genitalia:

"The pudendal's the nerve of love ... it innervates the pelvis from up above ... From its daring perch it makes sure you won't fall ... short of expectation's call ... or you won't be getting no love at all ..."

From such auspicious beginnings, our relationship lasted through our basic science years, into clinical rotations, until finally we got engaged after our third year of

medical school, and married four days before graduation. Any relationship that could withstand the battery
of a stressful medical education could probably withstand the test of time, we figured. And so we, too, joined
the statistics of medical students who found their mates
during training.

Gross Anatomy came and went, but not without me
being reminded quite personally that the bodies we
struggled over, learned from, dissected, and dreaded
were once people who lived and loved as we did. As my
own romance developed and deepened, I began to
imagine the lives of those whose bodies we worked on.
Who mourned them? Who dreamed of them? Who had
they been and wished to be? Who did they love? The
room was full of their shadows, and I had begun to feel
their weight. Yet, even as they made me recognize my
own mortality, they allowed me to fully enjoy my own
vitality.

In my childhood, I imagined the heart to be a velvety
valentine, lace-edged and gooey-sweet. During medical
school, I learned that the human heart is actually quite
difficult to uncover. If you are impatient or brutish, you
will dissect yourself into a mess. However, if you are patient and dissect very carefully, the layers will fall away in
even, smooth planes, and you will uncover a resilient
muscle, a fist-sized marvel of natural engineering. It is
not so mystical or mysterious as they make it in the
movies, just simple, beautiful, and alive.

War of the Worlds

When I was a little girl, the world was strictly divided in two spheres—the "outside" or American world, and "inside" or Indian one. My two worlds were divided by language, dress, custom, clothing, food, and most importantly, color. As a little brown girl growing up in the heart of the American Midwest, I was all too aware of the racial color line that marked my front doorstep. Verbal slurs, taunts in the schoolyard, and constant eyes upon myself and my family whenever we entered an all-white room were enough to make me aware of this dichotomy. I hated when my two worlds collided—when my mother, in her red bindi and bright cotton sari, would pick me up at school; when my little neighborhood friends would drop by unannounced and see my family eating a dinner of rice, daal, and fish with their hands. When these worlds stayed separate, however, all was right, and home was a safe, warm, protective place that smelled like chili peppers, felt like silks and jewels, and sounded like my parents' familiar voices.

When I grew older, and had to leave my parents' home for a college dormitory, I learned to take comfort in the safe spaces that other Indian Americans could afford me. They knew what it was like to be American during the week but Indian on the weekends, to pronounce and repronounce one's name for teachers who wondered why they couldn't just call you "Sue," to be accused of being a "cheeky American" by one's parents and a "nerdy Indian" by one's peers. With other Indian Americans, I learned to celebrate and love the skin I lived in. I learned to carry a piece of my safe, Indian home inside me even when I was in the big, bad, alien world.

When I arrived at Johns Hopkins Medical School, I was desperately in need of a familiar, brown face. Rita was it. It was moving day, and my stomach was churning with fear and anticipation as I pulled into the parking lot of our architecturally challenged medical school dormitory. It was only a few minutes later when my mother, who has an excellent cultural radar, exclaimed, "Look, here comes an Indian girl! She must be in your class!"

And so she was. We looked at each other and smiled with familiarity. Ah, our faces seemed to say, here's an anchor, here's a piece of home. That's not to say that Rita and I were ever that similar. Far from it. In fact, my overwhelming first impression of Rita was that she was tall. Much taller than me. Much taller, I had thought to myself at the time, than Indian women should be. And she was lithe, and lean, and muscular—an athlete; something else I was not. What kind of an Indian woman is this? I had wondered uncomfortably to myself, afraid that my potential slice of home would not fulfill some ridiculous cultural criteria.

I need not have worried. Rita was, if there is such a thing, as Indian as they come. She had recently spent time working at a hospital in South India, she informed me, where she had brushed up on her Tamil. Although I had been to my parents' home of Calcutta many times, working in an Indian hospital was still a dream of mine at that time. In fact, being able to "return" to India as a physician to help the poor was a philanthropic fantasy that I, like many other children of Indian immigrants, had carried to medical school. Later, when visiting Rita in her dorm room, I would see photos of her visit to India plastered all over her walls. In each and every picture, her long hair was oiled, braided, and wrapped in flower garlands. With her bright cotton saris and gold bangles, she was indistinguishable as an American. In that dorm room, I would listen to music, and drink wine, and eat her mother's leftover tupperwared *uppma* and *medhu vadai*. In that dorm room, I would feel secure, for in Rita I would find an Indian home away from home.

I still remember, that first moving day, she was wearing calf-length floral pedal pushers, a rather beat-up-looking "Harvard Track" sweatshirt, and the most enormous sneakers I had ever seen on the feet of an Indian woman. She shook my hand with a huge, toothy grin. I couldn't help but like her immediately.

Over the next two years, neither Rita's grin nor her wardrobe changed considerably. Although she was extraordinarily elegant when she wanted to be, she usually chose loose Indian-print cotton skirts or the ubiquitous pedal pushers. Sweatshirts and sneakers were a staple. So was her infectious sense of humor. Rita was my study buddy, but often, our study sessions would disintegrate into laughter, or manic food festivals.

Her illness started with a year-long cough that none of us thought anything of.

"Ahem, ahem," I had teased, imitating the dry cough that constantly interfered with our studies.

"Stop!" she had shouted. Although her high-pitched,

breathy laugh made her sound like Marilyn Monroe, the force at which she was pelting me with the balled-up sheets of notepaper and index cards reminded me that she was a serious athlete.

"Will you please go to University Health for that bronchitis?" I had asked sternly. I don't remember if she agreed. I wish now that I had been more insistent.

But neither I, nor Rita's other close friends, had given it another thought. Why should we? We were young and healthy, and the absolute worst thing in our lives was the upcoming pathology, or pharmacology, or physiology exam. Or so we thought.

"I have a terrible cramp in my leg," Rita complained one day as we were leaving the second-year lecture hall.

I hoisted my heavy bag to the floor and felt her leg amateurishly. I'm not sure I would have known enough to recognize something if I had felt it. But I hadn't.

"It must be because you've been practicing for your dance recital so much," I reasoned, referring to an upcoming Indian dance performance Rita was giving at the school. "Maybe you should chill out on the heavy practice schedule?"

I didn't pursue that either. In fact, I know that Rita continued her heavy practice schedule, even though her bronchitis seemed to be getting worse. It wasn't like Rita to be sick, or for that matter, to complain. But somehow, it didn't seem to register with me. I was stressed-out from second-year studies and assumed her exhaustion was a result of the same stress. I should have remembered how laid-back Rita was about her studies. I didn't.

The day of Rita's dance performance, everything seemed to go off beautifully. In her shining *Bharat Natyam* costume, her *kajal*-lined eyes dancing, her hands posed in classical *mudras*, Rita looked like a temple sculpture come to life. My heart tightened with pride at my culture displayed so gorgeously before the audience of my medical peers. But after the performance, Rita seemed exhausted, her normal jubilance dampened by what I assumed must be tiredness. I can still remember her breath catching in her throat as she panted, gasping for air a little longer than she should have.

A few weeks later, Rita came down with a horrible cold. "You really have got to take care of yourself, girl," I scolded when I came over, my arms full of missed notes and old tests. Our final exams were coming up, and it would be unthinkable for Rita to miss them. In her ill state, she studied at home. When she arrived to take the exam, I remember thinking how horrible she looked. But the dark circles under my own eyes didn't make me think Rita's appearance was anything unusual. Spring Break was coming up, and we all obviously needed a break. Medical school was brutal.

I arrived back from vacation to hear that Rita was in the hospital. She had suffered what looked like a stroke, possibly from an autoimmune disease. I rushed in to see her, but found her chipper as usual.

Despite the array of tubes and medical equipment all around her, Rita managed to let off an air of psychic, if not physical, health. She had covered the walls of her hospital room with beautiful batik prints and photographs of her family. On the side of her IV pump was a colorful picture of the plumply pleasant elephant-headed god, Ganesha.

It was the Indian imagery, more than anything, that reassured me. Rita was an intelligent, overachieving Indian American girl, just like me, and the worst thing

that happened to people like us was that we were for-
bidden from going to our proms, or got a "C" in school,
or had to dump our white boyfriends in fear of parental
disapproval. We were golden children. We were safe.

"I'm going to beat this thing," Rita had laughed, and I
had agreed. "I'm doing great at my physical therapy," she
practically gloated, gleefully demonstrating that she
could already squeeze and unsqueeze a rubber ball with
her paralyzed hand. She was an incongruous athlete, in
hospital gown and blue bedroom slippers.

"I think I'm going to sign up for the surgery rotation in
the fall," Rita had told me confidently. "I want to get it
out of the way."

Although I had some hesitation about her being able
to withstand the grueling surgery schedule, I had reasoned to myself that if she couldn't begin in the fall, she
could at least begin with surgery in the winter. Little did
we realize at the time she would not live beyond August.

Cancer.

It's an ominous word to me now, even though it had
never been. I was born after cancer had lost much of its
horror, and by the time I was in medical school, I had the
feeling that we were winning the war against the horrible
disease. My own grandmother, among numerous other
people I knew, had fought against cancer and won. When
I first heard Rita's diagnosis, I was under the assumption
that she would do the same. In fact, until the very end, it
had literally never entered my mind that she could die.
Rita was young, healthy, a vegetarian, a champion athlete, and a *Bharat Natyam* dancer. Most of all, she was
my friend, and it was utterly inconceivable to me that
anyone so young and successful could ever lose to this

conquerable disease. Cancer? It would be difficult, I thought, but Rita would beat it. Of course she would.

"That med student in your class, do you know her? The one with lung cancer," a resident had commented casually to me, and then continued, without waiting for an answer, "I saw her pathology slides today. She's in a really bad way. Awful, in fact. I've never seen malignancy like that."

Even then, I brushed it off. What did an idiot, insensitive resident know? I was new to the medical game, and was still enough of an outsider to be unaffected by such words. "The doctors," at that time, were still "other people." And this time, the doctors were obviously wrong.

Since Rita had fallen sick exactly at the end of our second year of medical school, the course of her illness occurred during my first clinical rotations in the hospital. Two months into her illness, I was doing pediatrics. Even when one of my first pediatric patients was a little five-year-old girl with terminal leukemia, I struggled to keep my work and personal psyches separate.

"There's something wrong with my blood," the little girl had explained to me. "But they're working on a cure now so that I can get better when I grow up."

As I read about my patient's disease, dutifully charting her vital signs, tracking her chemotherapy regimens, and reporting on her daily progress, I knew that the little girl was probably wrong. Although science was speedily working on cures for her disease, her prognosis was not good. My heart went out to the little girl and her family, and yet, I could not accept that their fate might also be mine.

I, like many other close friends and classmates, would

visit Rita in the evenings and on weekends, oftentimes still wearing my white coat and stethoscope to gain easy access to her room. Despite the costume, I left any medical personality I might have gained that day at the door. With Rita, there was no doubt in my mind that fate was on our side.

"She's getting better every day," Rita's mother would say waveringly to me, and I would wholeheartedly agree.

"She's so strong, Auntie," I would say confidently, squeezing her hand.

And yet, I was beginning to have an uneasy feeling. It was awful to see this woman, a typical Indian mother with long hair, gold hoop earrings, and a penchant for spicy food, as a permanent resident of the hospital. She puttered around the hallways of our teaching hospital, taking care of Rita, managing to eat some of the bland cafeteria fare herself. The expression on her face—firm, steadfast, determined—reminded me of looks I had seen on my own mother's face over a lifetime of childhood illnesses.

Once, on a train between Calcutta and Santiniketan, a man attempting to swing his heavy suitcase onto a high rack had dropped it directly on my ten-year-old head, knocking me more than a little dizzy. A split second later, I heard my mother's normally calm voice shrill with vicious anger. She spat angry words, like razors, at the man until he apologized profusely to both my mother and myself. The expression on her face was like that of a mother tiger defending her young. It was a similar expression I saw now on the face of Rita's mother. The ferocity on Auntie's face made me realize the situation was more serious than I was perhaps allowing myself to believe. This time, it wasn't a callous traveler she was fighting, but death itself.

The last time I saw Rita was before she was transferred from Johns Hopkins to a hospital in Boston, near her parents' home. Although it was my understanding that she was being transferred because she was getting stable, I wonder now if the Hopkins doctors had in fact lost hope. Rita had looked awful. Her frame, normally lithe and dancer-like, was frail and sickly-thin. Her shoulders, usually rounded and graceful, jutted out of her blue hospital gown like bony knobs. The Hickman catheter sticking out of her chest opened her gown a bit, so that I could see how visible her sternum and ribs had become. Her earthy brown skin had become yellowish, while her shiny black hair had fallen out in clumps, making it appear patchy beneath the flimsy paper cap on her head. Worst of all, her normally sparkling eyes were tired and dull. Darling Rita, whose infectious laugh had kept me going for two years of medical school, was too tired to smile. The sweetest thing is, she tried.

"Bye, Sci-Fi," she managed to say in a harsh whisper.

I felt my heart wrench at her silly nickname for me. "I'll come see you in Boston," I promised, kissing her papery, dry cheek.

She couldn't manage anything else, but was attacked by the fit of coughing that usually followed any attempt at speech. I held a cup to her lips. She spit out mucous and blood. I looked away, since I knew that she hated anyone, including her close friends, to see her when she was so ill. But Rita was too tired to care about that anymore either. I knew then that we might not have much time left.

We didn't. A few weeks after I saw her last, I got news of her death.

Recently, I attended a workshop for South Asian American women in Boston, Rita's hometown. As it is with Indian communities, two other women at the workshop knew Rita or her family. Early one morning, on a rooftop garden overlooking Rita's alma mater, we talked about my colleague, my friend, my sister. They sat in a circle around me, twelve teary-eyed brown faces, and re-created some sense of "inside" world for me.

"If we don't mourn her, who will?" blurted out a young woman, her East Coast twang and brusque manner belying her traditional Indian face and long dark hair. "She was one of us. She was one of us."

As I continue my medical career without Rita, I take each step tentatively. Every time I see someone with lung cancer, or meet a dying young person, or hear a patient with a dry, hacking cough, it shakes me. I see Rita's face suddenly, unpredictably as I walk the hospital corridors. Somewhere on the borderline between the worlds of doctors and patients, Indians and Americans, insiders and outsiders, Rita's memory lives for me.

This year, she would have graduated medical school.

In the Trenches:
The Clinical Years

If Med School Were Must–See TV

Thursday night. Ten o'clock. NBC. All over this great continent, people are easing their variously sized buns into their Naugahyde La-Z-Boy recliners, popping open sodas, diving into some chips, ready to have their spines tingled, hearts wrenched, and brains teased by their favorite must-see television drama. Its name? Of course, *ER*. And I, too, am sitting here, eyes glued to the boob tube. The one difference between me and the rest? (Besides my lack of recliner?) I, horror of horrors, actually can't stand America's favorite prime-time drama. In fact, as I watch, my hand is itching to change the channel. But for some reason, I can't. Am I doing some creative medical learning? Moved by the honor of my noble profession? Lusting after the way the male docs on the show fill out their scrubs? Hardly. I'm doing research. Or at least, that's what I'm telling myself.

They're so relaxed. That's the first thing that strikes me. OK, yeah, they emote an air of business, of stress, of the grim-lipped confidence to make life-and-death decisions. They furrow their brows, their eyes well up with tears, they bark out for normal saline with KCL, or five milligrams epi—"stat." But ultimately, they're completely and totally relaxed. They don't have bags under their eyes, they don't drink half as much coffee as any regular doctor, and they have way too much time to discuss their personal lives. (Way too much.)

I've never felt that relaxed in a hospital. Every time I walk into Hopkins, my stomach drops. It's silly, I know. I'm studying to be a doctor. But still, I hate hospitals. And the part of the hospital I hate most of all is the E.R. There are no windows. It smells. (Of vomit. Sweat. Excrement.) And the pace is far, far faster than anything my normal body clock can adjust to. A drunk here, a heart attack there, and interspersed in between, three vaginal bleeds, two drug overdoses, a kid with appendicitis, and an old homeless lady who thinks she sees Jesus in her trash bin. I never had as much fun as these folks on the TV show seem to. Then again, I hardly had the time (or opportunity) to flirt with George Clooney. Or even a George Clooney look-alike.

My emergency rotation was my first clinical experience in the hospital. And it was a doozy. When I informed my basic science professors of my choice, they looked at me strangely and said, "Great, I guess you'll jump in with both feet, huh?" It didn't help that my rotation was the first time the mandatory emergency clerkship was instituted at Hopkins. And so, the residents and attendings were just as raw at the teaching aspect of clinical medicine as we were at the learning part of it. I still remember my first day. It was the orientation lecture and I, typically, was late. I didn't think five minutes would make that much of a difference. Until I got lost in the bowels of the hospital basement, and five minutes became fifteen. The attending in charge of our four-week clerkship was describing an overhead transparency when I finally walked in.

As I squeezed myself into a chair, he looked pointedly at me and said, "And that comes to 'Must Not Do' rule number four: You must not be late to any conference, shift, or lecture without a preapproved valid excuse."

Needless to say, I hadn't preapproved my misguided sense of direction. It was an ominous way to start my clinical career.

There are few medical students on *ER*. The one who was there, John Carter, is now a resident. Even before he graduated, however, one never really got the sense that he was in school. He went to no lectures, took no tests, didn't really seem to have any requirements, and certainly didn't follow a group of "Must Not Do" rules. In fact, he was pretty much cut loose, allowed to play doctor in an emergency room playground. Oddly enough, he also had very few other classmates. When I was in the emergency room, it was swarming with medical students each trying to one-up each other. Ultimately, our main difference with Carter is that we left. He, it seems, not only had no "Must Not Do" rules, but a contract that extended beyond one season.

But the problem I have with *ER* is more than my lack of empathy for Carter—it's in the show's utter incongruity with my own experience in emergency medicine. OK, the show is obviously not real life, but an easy way in which I can point that out is to utilize, as I remember it, that well-meaning but anal-retentive emergency medicine attending's list of no-nos (which I was late for):

Must Not Do Rule 1: You must not forget to introduce yourself to each and every person on a shift. On *ER*, there are only about ten people who seem to day in and day out cover a major urban emergency room. There's no one to introduce yourself to because no one goes home. In real life, not introducing oneself, particularly to nurses, nursing aides, and other paramedical professionals, may result in them thinking you are an upstart medical student snob and making your life a living hell. It's not easy to do one's clinical duties when there's an underground conspiracy against you. I remember one pompous classmate who made the mistake of ordering around some of the emergency nurses. He couldn't figure out why, for the rest of the month, he was getting stuck with patients who would as likely as not vomit on his shoes.

Must Not Do Rule 2: You must not write directly in the chart. "I will not have any lawsuits brought against this hospital because of a medical student mistake," our emergency medicine attending had told us. Feeling like utter fools, we wrote out our notes on scrap paper, only to have our residents rewrite the entire history and physical again, instead of merely correcting and co-signing it, as they would on other services. On *E.R.*, I never saw John Carter having to turn in his histories like some poor-handwriting-plagued grammar schooler. Did that guy ever get treated like the peon that a medical student is?

Must Not Do Rule 3: You must not abbreviate. No kidding. Despite the fact that abbreviations are the heart and soul of the medical note—A "76 y.o. LOL c̄ a h/o MI, HTN, DM, CVA, CABG, MVA" is, in English, a very unfortunate seventy-six-year-old little old lady with a history of myocardial infarction, hypertension, diabetes mellitus, stroke, bypass surgery, and a motor vehicle accident—we poor underlings in the emergency dungeon were required to write out longhand phrases like "head, ears, eyes, nose, and throat exam" which, as every medical student knows, is "HEENT." The docs on TV seem to live, eat, and breathe cool-sounding abbreviations. They also really like medico-sounding phrases like "Come on, people, let's move!" and, the ever-popular, "Stat!" (which, interestingly enough, I have never heard spoken out loud during my entire medical training).

Must Not Do Rule 4: You must not be late to any conference, shifts, or lectures without a preapproved valid excuse. I know timeliness is next to godliness (and godliness is next to being a doctor), but it is just in my personality to be perennially running late. Worse still was Dr. Rahaman, a rather arrogant Indian surgical resident rotating through the emergency department when I was. The first time I attended sign-out rounds (at change of shift, when the old group of doctors describes the patients remaining on the floor to the new group of doctors), Dr. Rahaman was embarrassingly late. Worse still, he strolled in with a calm air of assurance. The attending running rounds had bellowed, "Dr. Rahaman, I will remind you that rounds start at seven, not seven-thirty! Next time, I'll have you kicked out of this residency program! Is that clear?" While I was quaking, Dr. Rahaman had merely grinned superciliously, assured that a surgeon could not be harmed by a lowly emergency doc. (Here *ER* is not off the mark. The show's surgeon Peter Benton is pretty accurately arrogant.) I've never seen such a scene on *ER*, where everyone seems to run perennially late too. Maybe that's because coming in late on TV seems to be the badge of honor that says, "Look at me! I didn't sleep alone last night!"

Must Not Do Rule 5: You must not perform any procedures you have not first seen. "See one, do one, teach one." That's the medical student motto. On *E.R.*, the star medical-student-turned-resident, John Carter, always seems to jump right over the first stage and intubate, cardiovert, and otherwise perform dramatic lifesaving procedures. I know it's TV, but it's just not realistic. As a woman, I had to actually struggle to do procedures during my emergency clerkship. Perhaps that was because Dr. Rahaman, that same pompous surgeon who had been scolded at rounds, took some particular interest in dictating to me during my rotation. While he let the male medical students try many different procedures for the first time, he gave me a hard time about sewing up even a simple laceration. "Have you been practicing your stitches?" he would singsong to me annoyingly. "You can't sew if you haven't been practicing your stitches!" He made it sound like I was a truant home-ec student rather than a doctor-in-training. And where was I supposed to be practicing my stitches, if not with patients? On his mouth? I felt like I was back in grade school, and convincing my resident to let me do a procedure was almost as impossible as convincing my sexist gym teacher to let the girls bat in softball.

Must Not Do Rule 6: You must not perform any procedures without appropriate supervision. OK, on *E.R.*, that stereotypically competitive Asian woman medical student did almost kill somebody by not following this rule. But how many times has John Carter swept into a room and performed some complicated procedure without supervision? Lots. And he didn't have to contend with a Dr. Rahaman.

Must Not Do Rule 7: You must not introduce yourself as "doctor." On other rotations, my superiors would introduce me as "Doctor DasGupta" even if I was uncomfortable with it. But being prohibited from doing so only made me feel like an utter nincompoop. The mere words "student doctor" conjures up notions of experimentation in an impoverished and suspicious community already convinced that big bad Johns Hopkins is using inner-city patients as laboratory rats. And inevitably, the words "medical student" would make people ask, "Oh, you're studying to be a nurse?"

Must Not Do Rule 8: You must not violate patient confidentiality. I suppose there's nothing as unconfidential as national TV, but even still, on *E.R.* they are constantly discussing patients in elevators, open hallways, and work stations. It's a mistake we make in the real-life hospital too, but get burned for. Dr. Rahaman, for instance (my favorite bad resident), was once loudly telling me about a rather aromatic alcoholic patient when he turned around and began shouting, "Where is my smelly guy? Where's that smelly guy?" I didn't know how to tell him the patient was standing right behind him.

Must Not Do Rule 9: You must not disrespect patients. On *E.R.*, they never seem to resent patients the way real doctors do in the hospital. While that's commendable, it's not very real. On TV, for instance, they rarely use the phrase that is so often applied to elderly, decrepit, but really not emergently ill patients who so often crowd waiting rooms in the middle of the night: GOMER—which stands for "Get out of my E.R.!"

Must Not Do Rule 10: You must not use the acronym "E.R." On the hospital totem pole, emergency docs not only practice in the hospital bowels, they reside there. They're considered (at least by some internists) to be physicians who practice cookbook medicine (if A happens, do B; if C happens, do D) in a one-room dungeon. To combat this notion, and perhaps to distance themselves from must-see TV, the emergency physicians at Hopkins insisted that we call the E.R. the E.D., or emergency department. Unfortunately, it just couldn't stick, and even attending physicians would slip and use the blasphemous abbreviation. Ultimately, it's like the television phrase "daytime drama"—the folks at the network may want us to use it, but a "soap opera" by any other name is still as histrionic. And the E.R., by any other name, still smells like puke.

I have a recurring fantasy about the show *ER.* In it, I and a couple of other crazed, beleaguered medical students take over a live taping with ouzies (still dressed, of course, in our short white coats) and demand that the actors play out a realistic script of our own creation. In it, John Carter would be basely humiliated, George Clooney exposed as a vain airhead who got his degree in the mail, and none of the women on the show would be allowed to wash their hair or put on makeup (hospital realism has its price). There would be fewer exciting cases, more drudgery, less cardioversions, more paperwork, less sex, more frustration. Of course, now that I think about it, the show would be pretty awful and horribly boring. Why should people turn on the tube to watch something they can go in to work to see?

I suppose there's a lesson to be learned from the fact that *E.R.* was created by Michael Crichton, a frustrated medical student who graduated from Harvard Medical School but never went on to do a residency. "It was too stifling, and not at all creative," I once heard Crichton say about medicine on a late-night talk show. Kind of ironic that he's filling America's imagination about the thrill of a profession he was too bored to remain in.

In response to the medical school adage "see one, do one, teach one," I often quip, "Those who cannot do, teach." I suppose that's kind of like *E.R.* Those who can't be doctors play them on TV. Those who can't be actors watch those who can't be doctors play them on TV. And those who can't bear to even watch, write for prime time.

Hey, anyone know the number of Michael Crichton's agent?

A Boy

This is a letter to a boy who died that night under the streetlight.

This is a letter to a boy whose eyes were wide open, staring straight up into the night, into the light. No one bothered to close them.

This is a letter to a boy whose back was muscular and broad; whose skin was dark and smooth. Perfect, healthy, young. All but for the big round hole in his chest. The size of a silver dollar.

This is a letter to a boy whose blood flowed down streets never touched by milk and honey (it's the street in front of the projects, the one that runs down to the city jail). It was like wet tar on the pavement, dark shadows under the too-bright light.

This is a letter to a boy I see not with my own eyes, but with the eyes of a man I think I love. He tells me, over and over, about your face, and so, I see you more clearly than he does anymore. He's gone running now, trying to erase your image from his mind. He doesn't know I've got it in mine.

This is a letter to a boy who died before his eyes. He saw you die under the streetlight, rivers of blood flowing down streets not paved with gold, eyes open, scorched by the overhead sun (courtesy of Baltimore Gas and Electric). His eyes, too, burned from the sight of you. He keeps rubbing them, as I rub his back. He cried over you, and that made me love him.

Is that horrible?

This is a letter to a boy who died in a drive-by, or over a drug deal, or because his stupid friend decided to be cool and wave his drug-dealin' big brother's gun around. I don't remember him telling me why you died. I don't think he can remember. All he remembers is seeing you under that streetlight, wet in the growing pool of your blood. Your back beautiful and broad. Bare-chested, muscles like those of a statue we stood in line to see in Florence. Your face, he says, just looked as though you were sleeping. With your eyes open? I don't know, that's what he said.

This is a letter to a boy who died before another boy's eyes. You were black and he was (still is) white, and even though that mere fact usually makes it a good story, that's not really the point. Well, not so much. The white boy, you see, had gone to school in the inner city, a school where (unlike in the world) he was an utter minority. He was called "Shorty," and jumped in the parking lot a couple of times, and knew when to look behind him, and knew when to run. He was on the soccer team, and was good, but not good enough to get respect. Not good enough to stop people from beating him up. And even though, at his ten-year high school reunion, he heard that a couple of old friends had been killed by guns, he'd never seen someone who died because of one. You were the first.

He was on an ambulance ride. He was on an ambulance ride. He was on an ambulance ride. And then, the sirens went off.

A call came in. A call came. A call.

Static, noise, adrenaline, excitement. His first night with the macho-macho ambulance guys. He wanted to make friends with them. He wanted to go out for a beer after the night was through. He didn't want them to think he was a med student snob. He didn't want them to think he didn't respect their work. He didn't want them to think he was only there as part of his emergency rotation. He wanted them to like him.

This is a letter to a boy who died the night another boy was making plans to go out for a beer with some new friends. They were just about to go, too, when the call came in. And the sirens went off.

Bumpety bump. Swerve and dash. Over every Baltimore pothole not for the need but to give the boy in back a thrill. To show their importance. To shake him up a little. But he didn't mind. Sitting in the back with the stretcher and the IV tubing and the orange emergency kits, he was excited. It was fast-fast. More so than med school could ever be. Like a rock-and-roll roller coaster. It was an adventure.

Bump. Some tubing fell on him, entangling him like so many sexy snakes. Bump. Or sirens, with their promises and songs, luring him to his doom. Bump. A siren song not of temptation, but of rescue. Not lured to his doom, but rescuing another from it. Very sexy, to be a macho-macho paramedic guy.

The dudes up front were calling back to him: "Boris, you still hangin' in there, man?" Their voices were smiling and deep.

He said he was. He liked them. He wanted them to like him.

This is a letter to a boy who was dying when the call

came in, and another boy who went bumpety bump, swerve and siren, to rescue, to save, to be sexy. The same thing as gangbanging, since boys do that, too, to be sexy. To sing their macho siren song, luring others to their doom even as they themselves escape. The ambulance dudes weren't that different. It's the same thing as gang-banging, just the flip side. Like cops and robbers, gang-bangers and paramedics. The ones who bleed, the ones who bandage. There but for the grace of God, and all that. A little yin-yangy.

This is a letter to a boy who went and a boy who came.

This is a letter to a boy who was lying there, so still, when the ambulance pulled up.

The dudes were up and at 'em. Running, leaping, orange boxing. But the boy along for the ride just stood there. Watching the halo of streetlight illuminating everything like a play.

"Boris," they called.

But he was thinking, I guess that's it. No beer tonight. No beer for this kid. Lying in his own blood.

"Boris," they called.

I guess that's it.

This is a letter. A lett. This is. This.

One boy, two boy, rich boy, poor boy, white boy, black boy, run, run, run.

When he would hear footsteps behind him in high school, he wouldn't turn around. He would just run like he was going for that big soccer goal, that goal that would make him a hero, that goal that would make him stop getting beat up, that goal that would make all the girls clap for him. He would run, run, run. And sometimes, he would get away.

Not today.

This is a letter to a boy who didn't get away. Well, two.

That night, there was crying. A mother, a brother, an uncle, a homie or two. That night, there was crying. A live boy who didn't know the dead one. A live boy who made a girl cry too.

This is a letter for the living and the dead, for the tears, for the blood on the pavement.

Lamplight, streetlight, bulb light, sun. Let them illuminate the dark corners. Let them protect all the mothers' sons. There is a warm boy in my arms, but the arms of another woman are cold.

This is a letter. This is a letter. This is a letter.

With no one to send it to.

Song of the Dying Ova

It's the dilemma of all young, professional women, I suppose. How, where, *when* to fit the mystical process of reproduction into the unerringly practical cycle of our professional production. It's the call of success versus the bleatings of our unfertilized ova as they plummet to their doom. As a woman in her mid-twenties entering the good-old-boys profession of medicine, I've come to realize that the more entrenched I become in my training, the louder those bleatings get. In fact, much to my boyfriend's chagrin, the cries of my dying eggs had become almost deafening during the months I completed my rotation through the field of pediatrics.

Taking care of other people's children is actually a mixed blessing for a mamma-wanna-be like myself. Even though many of the mothers I meet are my age and younger, the fact that I have not had children makes giving parenting advice an awkward and often ridiculous undertaking. "You mean, you do all that with your kids?" asked one young mother incredulously after I barraged her with intricate, and perhaps impossible, parenting tips I had read about only moments before seeing her child. When I told her that, in fact, I did not have any children of my own, her face cleared. "No wonder," she blurted out with relief.

I had always thought I would have children by now. My own mother was twenty-one when she had me, and carted me around throughout her education, from undergraduate through Ph.D. She was lucky enough to have the flexibility to sit me next to her in classes, or leave me to play in the graduate student offices with other doctoral candidates in search of distraction. As I grew older, we grew more like close friends, sisters, than mere mother and daughter. Our proximities in age and our inseparability forged a bond closer than nannies and baby-sitters could ever allow. It's a pattern that's not really replicable in the world of medicine. Getting beeped to have your baby-sitter tell you that your child spoke her first word is not really the same as being there. I remember a female pathology professor of mine grumbling about not being able to understand what her children were saying anymore. This wasn't, as I had first guessed, due to some generation gap, but because her children were more comfortable speaking Spanish, the mother tongue of their nanny, than speaking English with their own mother.

While my fascination with motherhood probably stems from the tick-tock of the same biologic clock that beats out a rhythm in most American professional women, it also originates from my heritage. As a daughter of Indian immigrants, I come from a culture that venerates motherhood above all else. Bengal, the region of India from which my parents originate, is actually one of the few places in the world where goddesses still reign supreme, and mothers, earthly equivalents of the great goddesses, play a central cultural role. For example, when Indira Gandhi was prime minister, the most popular street graffiti in Calcutta portrayed "Mother Indira" as "Mother India"—dressed as the warrior goddess Durga, riding a fearsome lion, brandishing a sword against all demonic and parliamentarian foes. The image puts American icons of apple-pie-ness to shame. It's like Donna Reed meeting Mom-Zilla.

So, while these primal forces of procreation are making images of babies dance in my head, ironic fate places me in a pediatric ward. It's the perfect torture for fertility-minded women: make them take care of children all day while constantly reminding them of how much more training they must endure before having any of their own. Indeed, during the mornings, after our predominantly female team of doctors had left their own sleeping children to make rounds through the ward, we would catch families at their most vulnerable. Mothers sleeping in the C-shaped posture of protectiveness while their tubed, monitored, and IV-ed children slumbered in the nest of their arms. When we drew blood from or placed IVs in our pediatric patients, it was often the mothers who cried out in empathetic pain as their children's skin was pierced. It's more than a symbiotic relationship, I realized. These were people who used to inhabit one body.

It was also the discrepancies I saw among parenting that broke my heart. A child is a child is a child. Or so I used to think. Yet, two little girls named Trina and Michelle taught me otherwise. Both were five years old, both robed in the animal-patterned bright yellow robes of the pediatric ward. Beyond these superficial similarities, the two girls might have been from different planets. Trina, abandoned by her drug-addict mother, was suf-

fering from impetigo—eczema that had become super-
infected due to improper hygiene and neglect. Across
the hall was Michelle, diagnosed with a much more serious condition—a new-onset severe seizure disorder.
Despite the seriousness of her condition, however, the
little girl was bright, secure, and entertaining, chattering
away enthusiastically to anyone who would listen. While
Trina was old before her time, a small body with the em-
bittered face of an ancient crone, Michelle was wide-
eyed and trusting—the curly-haired epitome of innocent
childhood. The same day that Trina struck and cursed at
a nurse in the hallway, screaming, "Get the hell away
from me, you fucking bitch," Michelle and her mother
tripped by happily through the hallway. While one child-
ish voice screamed in outrage and anger, another sang,
"Skip, skip, skip to my lou. Skip, skip, skip to my lou. Skip
to my lou my darling."

Medicine, like raising children, is hard work, demanding toil, frustration, and heart. As more women enter the
field, it will not be acceptable anymore to penalize a
pregnant resident who takes maternity leave, look down
upon a physician who is late because her child is ill, or
equate a good doctor with one who cares more about
her patients than her personal life. Indeed, as more pregnant senior residents waddle around the hospital, making major medical decisions with extra large scrubs tied
around their protuberant bellies, younger women like
myself are gaining role models to look to and learn from.

There were no women with children in my medical
school class. However, in the classes below me, there appear to be more and more women who are both mothers
and future physicians. I recently saw a woman I know in
the hospital, dressed in the requisite white coat, with a

stethoscope around her neck, her pockets bulging with papers, tongue depressors, gauze, and the bevy of other medical goodies. There was one difference, however, because besides all of her medical equipment, she also had a baby strapped to her back. Although her husband was to shortly pick up the child, it was encouraging to see a medical student who was more than just a nervous trainee eager to please. Clearly, the times are changing.

While I look forward to the day I can combine motherhood and medicine, the song of the dying ova continues. It's actually got a pretty good beat. And the beat goes on.

What Bad Boys Will Be

I used to think the phrase was a bunch of patriarchal retro-macho huey. But taking care of teenagers of the male persuasion taught me that the idea has its own truism: boys, as they say, will be boys. I have my own addendum to that idea as well, which is: bad boys will be bad boys. Indeed, no matter where, when, or how, naughty little men will find one another and congregate. Even, it seems, in the hospital.

And so, we find an answer to that perennial television question—Bad boys, bad boys, what you gonna do? What you gonna do when they come for you?

The answer? Why, run to the hospital.

It's a Friday afternoon on the adolescent ward, and everyone is itching to go home. The residents are frantically finishing their work, the majority of patients are trying to convince their doctors that they really are well enough—cough, cough—to go home, but there are a roomful of patients, the boys in the back, we call them, who aren't all that eager to go; who are, in fact, busy trying to convince us that they are sick enough to stay.

Travis is a seventeen-year-old streetwise wisecracker. He sleeps, each morning when I come to examine him, with his mouth wide open, snoring deafeningly and drooling inelegantly upon his hospital pillow. He is curled up on his side, his childlike expression in direct contradiction to the drug trade he engages in when he is not in the hospital. I poke and prod at the shoulder which is, or so he says, in sickle-cell crisis so severe that he has to be admitted to the hospital for intramuscular Demerol injections. He doesn't wake up. When I finally do manage to rouse him, he peers up at me, blinking, through sleep-goo-encrusted eyes, an utter babe in the woods. Then he remembers. He pauses for a dramatic moment and lets out a heartfelt scream. It is terrible, and unconvincing. I think about lending him money for acting lessons.

Antonio is an eighteen-year-old pretty boy. He's also probably got some drug action going on, but he's got to split up his time with the ladies too. Last time Antonio was on the floor he was caught in the bathroom with another patient's mother. And they weren't chatting about politics. His sickle-cell crises tend to come in synchrony with Travis's. I think they probably don't get a chance to hang out so much at home.

Sean is a twenty-year-old paraplegic. They let him stay on the pediatric floor instead of shipping him off to an adult unit basically because the pediatrics department is about the only family he's had since he had his spinal cord blown out during a drive-by at the age of thirteen. His homies apparently used to come and give him lots of support, but in the last few years they've tended to lose interest. His wheelchair makes him too much of a liability on the street. Bone infections from repeated bed sores make him too sickly to be much fun. Now he mostly tortures nurses on the adolescent floor. On his last admission, he threw a telephone at a head nurse who was taking too long to come and change his diaper. It's a bit different from his gangbanging days. Legend has it that he is always given his own room so that he can smoke pot with the tacit approval of the pediatrics department. My nose tells me that the legends might actually be true.

That afternoon, the boys in the back are hangin' out. Along with our three regular players are Antonio's latest girlfriend, Tiffany, who is not, as far as I know, anybody's mother, and Patrick, a small-for-his-age fourteen-year-old with a congenital deformity that gives him a stiff, unmovable webbed neck. I guess the fact that he can't turn away makes him a pretty good listener. And this afternoon, he is listening intently, because there is a performance going on. Antonio, beautiful, dramatic, in his undershirt and plaid boxer shorts, showing off his muscular body and Chinese character tattoos dancing over his biceps, is giving a lecture. Gathered around are his adoring fans, stiff-necked Patrick, sleepy-eyed Travis, and anxious Sean who is wheeling around Antonio in circles, all but popping wheelies.

"Listen, son," Antonio is saying generously, "I'm tellin' you the truth." A reclining Tiffany, busy gluing rhinestones on her nails, calls back her support, "Yes, you are."

Antonio recognizes her comment with a silent incline of his head, but keeps his eyes on his fellow men. "You hear what I'm sayin' son? You hear what I'm sayin'?"

Patrick, nervous and doubtful, is unable to either nod or shake his head. "Uh-huh," he mumbles, his eyes on the floor.

Sean doesn't allow his disability to hamper his disbelief. "Naw, son," he spits out, spinning his chair around Tonio for effect, "that ain't right. That ain't right. You tawkin' shit!" He's noticed I'm in the room and says the word "shit" as a voluble exclamation. I return his challenging look dryly but say nothing. I'm waiting to figure out what Tonio is saying that has gotten everyone so excited.

Travis, eyeing Tiffany out of the corner of a droopy eye, asks, "Tonio, man, you sure about what you're sayin'?"

The Chinese characters ripple as Antonio flexes his arms above his head for extra effect. "As sure as I am a one-hundred-percent-beautiful black man," he swaggers, grinning at his girlfriend.

She grins back.

But Sean pops his bubble. "Shit, man, you ain't black, you Puerto Rican."

Tonio's beautiful smile doesn't falter. "But ain't we all brothers?"

Sean wheels straight at him, his chair an extension of his aggression. "All that shit you been talkin', it ain't right, man, it ain't right."

My curiosity is utterly piqued. Drug trafficking technique? Sexual positions for multiple partners? New ways to assault nursing staff? What is it that Tonio has everyone so riled up about?

Then, the truth is revealed. Antonio strides side to side in front of the window, a lecturing professor before his blackboard of the world. "It's true, son, the continents—they weren't always like they are now," he announces, his tone a celebration. "They came apart because of somethin' real strong." He puts out both arms in a rapperlike gesture, crossing them stylistically over his chest. "It's called Teutonics!" he concludes gloriously.

Travis is too lazy to continue disagreeing. "Are you sure about that, man? That sounds crazy, man! The continents just moved apart like that?" Then, to himself, he mutters, "Man!"

But Sean isn't convinced. "Teutonics? I ain't never heard'a no Too-taw-nics, son." He adds the last word as an afterthought, and it punctuates his angry expression. He may be only borrowing Antonio's colorful words, but he looks like he would like more to borrow his healthy body. He wheels quickly over to me.

"You heard about this shit, Doc?"

Before I have a chance to answer Sean's question, however, Patrick pipes up unexpectedly from his bed. "Yeah, yeah, I heard of that. Teutonics. Yeah." Sean's look dries up his voice so that the last "yeah" is nothing more than a swallowed whisper.

The professor needs no more support than that. "It's like this, son." I notice that Antonio is addressing himself almost directly to Sean. While he knows that Sean isn't a real challenge to his authority, I guess Tonio can't stand not being liked by anyone. "The continents, you see, used to be all together in one big country. But then, they like slipped away from each other because of Teutonics."

"Uh-huh, that's right." This time Tiffany's call and response comes with a raised hand. She almost says, "hallelujah!" I change my mind. Antonio is more like a preacher than a professor.

"So Africa, you see, son"— his arms are moving expressively now, and he uses his dancer's body to illustrate his point—"Africa says to Europe, it says"—he holds up a stop sign with his hand—" 'Nigga, I don't want to be with you anymore.' And shit, son, Africa just took herself up and slipped right away."

I could let all the *shits* go, but I couldn't really let this one slide by me like some moody continent. "Antonio," I start to say, "come on, now."

But no one hears me over all the excitement.

"Africa just up and did that like that?" The impact of "teutonics" has awoken Travis from his droopy-eyed state. "Africa just up and said, 'I'm outa here'?"

"You better believe it, son," Antonio agrees.

"Like he says, like he says," Tiffany chimes in.

The momentum catches Sean and he pulls a three-sixty with his mood as well as his chair. "Too-taw-nics, man!" He says the word like he's cheering his favorite basketball team. "Too-taw-nics!" I guess he's decided to join the winning side. "Oh, yeah, oh, yeah, son, Africa just said to Europe, 'Lata', nigga! Lata'!' "

Patrick, too low for anyone else but me to hear, pipes in, "Later!"

The room bursts with energy like somebody scored a winning point. Sean's spinning around like some wheelchair bound Evel Knievel, Tiffany leaps up to put her arms around a strutting Antonio, and even sleepy Travis does an arms-in-the-air "whoop-whoop."

"Lata', son!" Antonio is shouting, "Lata', nigga!"

This is my chance. "Now Antonio," I say loud enough to be heard above the melee, "you're a very eloquent guy—"

"Whas' that mean?" challenges Sean from his chair. I guess he's wondering if I'm bustin' on his homie.

Antonio is looking at me quizzically. "Do you know what that means, Tonio?" I ask, and at his almost imperceptible headshake, add, "It means I think you're a good speaker."

He puffs up like the proud crow he is. "Oh, yeah, yeah, son, you hear that? Doc thinks I'm a public speaker, man! A fuckin' public speaker! That's phat!"

"Yeah, son, a public speaker!" Sean echoes.

"Which is why," I try to reclaim some ground, "I'm sure you can explain about plate tectonics without using words that might offend people."

He looks at me quizzically.

"Doc means since you Puerto Rican, you shouldn't be callin' all us niggas niggas," Travis pipes up cheerfully.

Oh, God. How to recover from that? "Not exactly," I start.

"That's cool, Doc, that's cool," Tonio is saying over me. "I don't have to call these niggas niggas."

"Tonio," I say warningly.

The boys burst out laughing. I can't stop from laughing myself.

It's quite a long way from Racism 101 at my Ivy League activist campus, not to mention Introduction to Geography, but this classroom I am lucky enough to witness is many thousands of miles away from any physical campus. I guess the most ironic part is that the word that describes Tonio's scientific discovery, "Teutonics," or Germanic culture, is even further away from these boys' reality.

They're dancing around the room now. Tonio and Tiffany are plastered against each other, doing the intercontinental grind, Travis is doing the tectonic stomp, and Sean is actually giving Patrick an around-the-world tour on the armrests of his wheelchair.

"Come on, guys!" I shout warningly, but they pull me into their fray. I don't resist too much.

I can feel the plates shift under my feet. And continents, cultures, worlds continue to slip and slide away from each other, and then back together again.

Boys, after all, no matter where you be, are just boys.

Of Mini–Moms and Misunderstandings

When I first moved to Baltimore, one of the first things I noticed—before the Inner Harbor, before the delicious crab cakes, before the middle-of-the-night gunshots—was a very unusual billboard that had even greater prominence beside Baltimore highways than the now dishonored Joe Camel. It read, "Virgin: Teach Your Kids It's Not a Dirty Word."

At first, I thought it was a good idea. Since it was an interest in public health, particularly adolescent health, reproduction, and contraception, that brought me to medical school in the first place, I was particularly struck by the Campaign for Our Children's "virgin" series. But something didn't sit well with me. Would teaching teens to embrace the word "virgin" really convince them not to have sex?

The first baby I delivered in medical school was to a mother who was also a baby. She was fourteen, with no prenatal care, no idea of how many weeks along she was, and no real emotions playing across her stoic face. That is, until she was in active labor. Then, she screamed like a banshee for her mother. It was an odd sociological spectacle: my young patient kicking and screaming her way through contractions in ways Lamaze never intended, refusing like a petulant child to bear down, and demanding that we immediately relieve her body of its even younger charge. "Get it out right now!!" She was hollering, not unlike many other mothers. The difference is, she meant it. She sincerely expected us, the medical personnel, to miraculously deliver her baby despite the fact that she was less than willing to follow any instructions. Needless to say, the infant was delivered despite my patient's bad attitude. It being my first delivery, my nervousness was only compounded by the mother's frenetic screeches, her sudden, failed lunges off the delivery bed, her nonstop gutter-mouth cursing. I was relieved I didn't drop my little slippery charge; my rebellious child's child.

In this country, the issue of adolescent pregnancy is phrased, at best, as a "problem," at worst, as a "war." (Militarism commandeering women's bodies again, folks.) Another popular slogan, whose origin was made clear to me by my first delivery experience, is "children having children." At first, this language seemed to me not only appropriate, but powerful. It wasn't until after my third year of medical school, when I was in a family-planning class during my Masters of Public Health program, that I began to see the fundamental problems in the messages that we send to adolescents about sex. Many are based directly on fear. One poster, for example, shows a miserable-looking teen mom and declares, "Baby-sitter needed. 24 hours a day, 7 days a week." Another commercial depicts a little girl putting on makeup, with the ominous background commentary, "if you think having sex with a thirteen-year-old makes you a man, think again." Despite the fact that research clearly shows that fear techniques have limited effectiveness with young people, slogans like these continue to be popular. While the "virgin" series and other "just say no"-esque messages don't focus on fear, abstinence messages are also negative. And ultimately, the problem with negative messages is that they tell an age group developmentally obsessed with immediate gratification not *what* to do but what *not* to do. And *not* is a word to which few teens respond well.

When I think about these public health campaigns, I can't help but remember the various teenage parents I have met during my medical school rotations, and imagine what their reactions to our messages might be. I remember, for instance, the many angry-faced gang-color-wearing teenage dads I have met, who slouch lazily in delivery room chairs, chatting on cell phones with their homies while their girlfriends labor painfully beside them. I imagine they only laugh when they see posters declaring "What do you call a man who makes a baby, then flies the coop?" with a picture of a tennis-shoe-wearing chicken beneath the words. Life is hard for these kids, and it probably takes a heck of a lot more to affect them than a giant chicken.

Cognitively, adolescents are operating on a different set of assumptions. I remember a twenty-two-week-pregnant teen in premature labor, who was told that it was less than likely that her baby would be able to lead a normal life. After a long conversation, the caring neonatologist convinced her to decide against any lifesaving measures for the little preemie, since they would be nothing more than expensive, painful prolongations of the inevitable. Then the father showed up. With his pants halfway down his butt, a handkerchief knotted over his short braids, and the inevitable cell phone tucked in his jacket, he was the epitome of tough. He seemed oblivious to the mother of his child, whose bed was tilted upside down to try and slow labor, but got immediately on the phone to his buddies. He utterly ignored his surroundings until a resident rolled the ultrasound machine into the room. As she watched the scan of the patient's abdomen, the resident began to do something that I, the third-year medical student, considered utterly inappropriate. She began to point out various parts of the fetus to the patient and the now-attentive baby's father. "This is the face, the arms, the leg," she said, much to my horror. And then, worst of all, "Oh, and look, there is the little penis. It's a boy."

The atmosphere in the room immediately changed. With a tug on his dangerously low pants, the young man got quickly back on the phone to his friends. "I'm havin' a boy," he declared proudly. "Yeah, man, I'm gonna have a son." The resident, perhaps realizing the avalanche her revelation had created, scurried quietly out of the room. I watched helplessly as the patient happily decided to ask for every heroic measure possible to save her baby's life. Apparently, she had completely forgotten all the neonatologist's explanations as she was swept away in her ex-boyfriend's gender-biased enthusiasm. Typical teenagers, the two had convinced themselves that the baby would be all right, merely because they wanted it to be so. Bad things, teens think, always happen to others, not to them. It's that mentality that gets many teens pregnant. It's that mentality that made this particular patient spend thousands of the hospital's dollars to put a small infant through a long series of painful, pointless procedures, only to finally die anyway.

After such spectacles of immaturity, it is perhaps

tempting for adults to clap teenagers in chains, or at least not allow them to date until they are in their thirties. Since we can't feasibly do either of these things, we hopefully bombard teens with messages to be abstinent, and try to scare them into remaining so. Clearly this "see no evil–encourage no evil" philosophy is not exactly working. Whether we like it or not, many adolescents are going to have sex. What's important then, is not only to impress upon them the necessity of contraception, but to make it utterly and overwhelmingly accessible.

At the adolescent health clinic, it was standard operating procedure to stuff the pockets and pocketbooks of all sexually active teens with condoms, and to encourage the young women to adopt an appropriate form of birth control for their lifestyles. "Oh, great," young women would usually say, "could I have some more?" One explained to me, "I don't want to get pregnant, but when you're going at it, it's just not romantic to look for protection." My experience with these girls convinced me that the idea that inner-city adolescents actually want babies (to fulfill themselves, to feel important, to have unconditional love) is primarily a myth. Most of my patients' mindsets were more like a fatalistic Russian roulette—if it happens, it happens (but of course it won't, to me).

Whether or not adolescents desire pregnancy, the most critical factor in helping them make informed and positive decisions is, of course, education: My OB/Gyn and adolescent health experiences in fact have taught me how shockingly unaware most young people are about their bodies. "I think I got some kind of a drip," young men who end up having huge gonococcal infections usually mumble at the end of a routine physical.

Similarly, young women are often more than unaware of their sexually transmitted diseases. "I think I got some kind of a pimple or something down there," a young woman with the most horrible venereal warts I have ever seen initially warned me. It is furthermore utterly common for young women not to have the slightest clue how many weeks' pregnant they are. One fifteen-year-old at OB clinic convinced me that she was at the most four weeks' pregnant, since she missed only one period. When I examined her, I felt something round and hard in my hand. I assumed it must be her uterus, and that my young patient was about four weeks off of her approximate due date. When my attending did another exam, she explained to me what that small round thing I felt was. It was the baby's head. The young woman was more than twenty-nine weeks' pregnant, and could feasibly have delivered a healthy baby that very day.

The most blatant example of a young woman's lack of awareness about her own body is a teenager whose birth I attended as a third-year on OB/Gyn. Like the first young lady whose baby I had delivered, this patient had more than a bad attitude. When I asked her permission to enter the room, she screeched at me, "I don't care who you are, just tell this bitch to get her fucking hands off of me!" The patient aimed a painful-looking kick at the resident who was examining her, which landed, luckily, on her shoulder.

"Ma'am," the exasperated resident spat out, "we are trying to help you!" From her intonation, it seemed she was contemplating kicking the patient back. Instead, she sat back down on the stool to continue her exam.

"What are you *doing*?" the young patient shrieked in what seemed like very real bewilderment.

"I'm trying to examine you with my hand, ma'am," the resident ground out. "Like I explained, I'm trying to see how far along you are."

"Get that bitch to get her hands out of there!" the patient hollered at me. "Why is she touching me down there?" Then, sincerely confused, she sobbed, "Why are you touching me down there?"

It was clear our patient didn't have the first idea about where her baby was going to come from. That was confirmed a few hours later, when our young patient was ready to deliver. She kicked, she screamed, she hollered, and she cursed, cursed, cursed. And then, when the child was crowning, and we could see little tufts of the baby's curly brown hair, our young patient cried in utter horror, "Oh my God! The baby's comin' out of my butt! It's comin' out of my butt!"

It wasn't until much later that anyone on our medical team had the heart to correct her anatomic understanding.

Despite misconceptions, misunderstandings, and even misbehavior, the mini-moms (and dads) I encountered during medical school reinforced to me the importance of empathy, access, and ultimately, education. Perhaps it's time for a poster aimed at those of us who tsk-tsk at teenage pregnancy but refuse to give kids the straight facts: "Misinformation: teach your adults it is a dirty word."

The Face of a Woman

A few years ago, I saw a provocative movie called *Citizen Ruth*. In it, a homeless, dirty, crass, inhalant-sniffing (yet, ultimately endearing) small-town bum (Laura Dern) gets pregnant. Her decision whether or not to have an abortion becomes the bone of contention between the town's bouffanted, Bible-thumping pro-life group and a lesbian-dominated politically impassioned pro-choice contingent. Both sides, under the guise of protecting Ruth's interests, unabashedly wheedle, lecture, and bribe her, yanking her reproductive decision-making from private to public. As protest marches, political intrigues, and a frenzied media get into the act, it becomes clear that Ruth, as an individual, as a citizen, never existed at all. Just as her living situation, her drug habit, her freedom (from jail) is controlled by the state, her reproductive choices are controlled, alternately, by two equally abusive sides of a political argument. Her very private decision is in the hands of the group, community, and national public. Ultimately, Ruth, having miscarried and thus making the question of abortion moot anyway, pockets her bribe money and slips out, utterly ignored and forgotten by both sides of the politically zealous battle. She existed for them only as a symbol, not as an individual. *Citizen Ruth* puts a face to what is too often a faceless debate, pointing out that pro-choicers and pro-lifers are sometimes similar in over-looking women's individual needs.

I have always been actively, utterly, and passionately pro-choice. Indeed, I was raised in a household where feminism was mixed into my baby food, where political activity was as important a learning experience as high school and college classes. By the time I was a teenager, a couple of close friends had experienced unplanned and unwanted pregnancies. I cannot imagine what they would have done had abortion services not been available to them, if they had to disrupt their educations to carry a pregnancy to term, or worse still, if they had been forced to choose unsafe, unsterile, backstreet abortions. Yet, even by the time I went to medical school, determined to be an OB/Gyn and women's health advocate, abortion was primarily an intellectual issue, a political rallying point. It would soon become more than that.

As I write this essay, I am nervous. I am nervous because I don't want to give any ammunition to those opposed to a woman's right to choose an abortion. I am nervous because this is a volatile topic sparked by the slightest flame. I am nervous because this fundamental right is in such jeopardy that the slightest critique may be interpreted as an assault against it. Yet, I must write about what I've seen. I must be able to critique that which I still believe in.

The first time I observed an abortion was during my OB/Gyn rotation. I had to fight for even that opportunity. Because, perhaps, of the political fury surrounding it, pregnancy termination is not a part of the medical student OB/Gyn curriculum at my school. I was told to ask special permission from the residents at the private Hopkins affiliate hospital where I happened to be placed at the time. I guess I was lucky to at least have the opportunity. At other medical schools, where it is not even a service provided by the residency program, students don't have the option of choosing to observe abortions.

The answer I received when first asking about abortions was a shock. "I really don't think it's appropriate," grumbled the third-year resident who was in charge of the pregnancy termination clinic. "You know, this is a really sensitive issue, and I think, for reasons of confidentiality and all that, it's really not right to have someone else in the room."

I was floored. I was a student, not an ogler interested in sensational experiences. How could I learn to provide this critical service if no one was willing to teach me? If I did go into OB/Gyn, how could I be a good physician having never even observed one abortion? How could I know what my patients were going through? How could I call myself a women's advocate?

Yet there was a part of me that understood. Sharon, the resident who had rebuffed me, wasn't just the doctor providing abortions that month. She was the only resident in her class who was willing to provide the service at all. Her classmates had taken the option to refuse to provide abortions during their residency. Sharon was protectively guarding what was obviously a highly criticized service. Eventually, after a late-night heart-to-heart when Sharon and I were on call together, she seemed to change her mind about me. A few mornings later, I would accompany her to termination clinic.

I was surprised at what a quick procedure a first-trimester abortion is. The woman comes in, her history is verified, a few reassuring words are spoken, she places feet in the stirrups, her genital area is draped with sterile cloth, laminaria (dilating seaweed sticks that expand with body's moisture) are removed from the cervix and counted, and then the procedure is performed. Whether it's vacuum or hand-suction curettage, the effect is the same: a lot of blood and tissue are removed at first fairly painlessly followed by a final period of intense cramping as the uterus is utterly emptied.

An abortion is, basically, nothing more than any other surgical procedure I have observed. It's a minimally invasive, brief experience. That is, if the emotional, cultural, and political underpinnings are not considered.

I had more in-depth experience with abortion provision during my fourth year, when I did a special sub-internship in reproductive health. During this rotation, I worked with a progressive and internationally renowned physician who performed both first- and second-trimester abortions. I evaluated, examined, and counseled women in pre-termination clinic as well as assisted the attending physician during abortions. This experience deeply disturbed me and made clear to me the importance of changing the physical, psychological, and cultural environment in which most abortions take place.

The women, age distributed, oddly enough, in their late teens or late forties, were lined up in hospital chairs in the waiting/recovery area outside the procedure room. While the older women were usually stoic and reserved, the younger girls had a tendency to work each other up, sharing horror stories of "the way my girlfriend said it would be" and "how much it hurt last time" until many young patients were terrified beyond belief. The lack of privacy for post-procedure patients was horrifying as well. The sight of a prone patient, woozy with adrenaline and pain, made the faces of those women still waiting tense in fright. I could hardly stand the assembly-line spectacle, and would run into the procedure room as quickly as I could.

But there, the experience was even more stressful. The attending physician I was working with did not believe in giving the women sedatives or painkillers. "If a woman stays calm," he explained to me, "it is usually not a problem. But giving a woman painkillers dulls her senses, and it makes me uncomfortable to perform a procedure on a woman who is cognitively not all there. Besides which, why subject a patient to anesthetic if it's not necessary?"

It sounded logical enough. But the result was far more upsetting and dramatic than his dry explanation. "Oh, God, I can't stand the pain!" women would exclaim. "Please, please, oh, God . . . Mommy!" another woman in her mid-forties shrieked.

"Come on, come on, you're not working with me," the physician would bellow authoritatively from his end of the table if any woman wiggled out of range. "Scootch back down here. Come on, now, I'm holding up my end of the bargain, you've got to hold up yours."

I didn't think it was exactly a fair deal. My stomach wrenched, my heart pounded, my palms poured perspiration as I tried with all my might not to empathize too much with the patients, not to put myself in their place. But it was impossible. Each procedure made me near-dizzy with anguish.

The interesting thing is, however, reactions were not consistent across the board. Most of the women wept aloud, squeezing my proffered hand to a near pulp, and had a demoralized, tragic affect. However, one particular group of patients, Baltimore's newer Eastern European immigrant community, had a radically different reaction to having an abortion.

The few Eastern European women I saw were calm, pleasant, and bore only the degree of nervousness to be expected by a patient having an outpatient procedure. One woman, Tania, was extremely sweet, chatting and laughing with me about her rambunctious children, who were out in the waiting room with their father. "This is my third abortion," she explained in her halting English. "I cannot pay for, care for, any more babies. My two children are very, very naughty. They keep me busy." Although she winced and was obviously uncomfortable during the procedure, she left smiling, thanking us, and promising to use her birth control pills regularly from now on.

The explanation for her reaction is, of course, self-evident. Women like Tania come from countries where restrictive birth control policies, combined with exorbitant cost and lack of access, have made abortions a first-line method of family planning. While this is obviously an abominable medical phenomenon, it clearly demonstrates that the controversy around abortion in the U.S. is predominantly culturally constructed. It does not, of course, make abortion for women in these countries any less individual or personal. Just because many countries have placed the choice in the hands of necessity, or an oppressive government, doesn't mean that this deeply personal power should not be in women's hands.

It becomes critical, then, to examine each woman's personal experience within her own cultural context, as well as her own personal experience. For instance, while

Tania's cheery reactions did not alarm or sadden me, similar behavior in a woman from a different community would make me concerned.

"You OK, honey?" I asked a little street-sassy fourteen-year-old African American young woman one day. "Do you want to squeeze my hand?"

She looked at me incredulously, her face a hardened mask. "What for? I ain't scared. I done this before." She didn't utter a peep, but stared unseeingly at the ceiling, her hands folded over her chest. Only the spasmodic flexion of her feet in the stirrups, with their raggedly cut, electric blue–colored toenails, betrayed her emotion. I wondered what other kinds of treatment she had endured, placid-faced, staring at the ceiling. I was strongly inclined to shake that frozen look off her face.

"There, all done. It wasn't that bad, was it?" the attending would chirp cheerfully as exhausted women in undignified positions dragged themselves up and pulled themselves together. After each procedure day, I had to stifle the impulse to bash him in the back of the head with a bedpan. He, on the other hand, usually grinned like a Cheshire cat, proud of the fact that he was the sole practitioner in the hospital providing oftentimes grisly second-trimester abortions. He would glow, "I go where other doctors fear to tread."

This self-promoting physician was world famous for his liberal politics, his championing of women, his reproductive health savvy. Yet, when it came to interpersonal sensitivity, he was, to say the least, a jerk.

These experiences have brought me to realize that political progressiveness, lobbying for policies, or even working for women's advocacy is not enough. Indeed, abortion is an intensely personal experience. As health care providers, we must stalwartly protect the privacy, dignity, and emotions of our patients, and in doing so, protect our own privacy, dignity, and emotions as physicians.

My most poignant experience was doing a pre-termination exam on a woman in her mid-forties, old enough to be my mother. When I walked into the tiny exam room, the discrepancies in our ages made me initially nervous. I think they startled her as well. She stared at me, her face a bit hard, a bit wary. Adopting my best professional tones, I started going through her history. Eventually, I got to the part I was dreading to ask her.

"Now that I've explained the details and the potential risks," I said crisply, looking up from my paper, "you're . . . um . . ." I involuntarily softened my voice, "sure you want to have this procedure?"

She paused. Our interactions to that point had been very professional—question and answer. But my change in tone seemed to affect her. "I'm very sure," she said firmly. She added, with a thoughtful look at me, "My daughter is twenty-two." Four years younger than I was at that time. We smiled at each other, each having thought the same thing.

"We're so close, best friends. I'm the one who gives her lectures on responsibility and birth control." The woman brushed back her thick salt-and-pepper hair, laughing ruefully, "Now, how can I face her? I feel like such a fool." Tears brimmed brightly in her eyes.

I handed her a box of Kleenex, suddenly feeling my super-professional manner falling away, and my real personality emerging. It was her honesty that allowed us to interact as two women, older and younger, patient and physician, a mother and a daughter.

"I'm really close to my mother too," I said. "I don't think your daughter will think anything. Especially if you're close. I think she will welcome the chance to support you." I was speaking from my heart, because in this older woman, I could easily see my mother's face.

"I know," she grinned through her tears. "I'm just embarrassed. I thought I had reached menopause, but I obviously haven't." I nodded. It was common enough. Her smile soon crumbled again. "I used to have all the answers, but I guess I don't. I feel terrible about myself."

I couldn't help myself from tearing up too. "Oh, no," she laughed waterily, "now you're crying."

"I really hope," I said sincerely, "that you don't beat yourself up about this. Things happen, you know. I for one don't think you're irresponsible at all. You're making the responsible choice given your life situation. It's not like you're taking it lightly." I dabbed my own eyes with a little embarrassment. "You know, daughters understand that mothers aren't infallible either."

She thought about this for a moment. "Thank you," she said lightly, then, taking my hand, she said gently, "Now, shouldn't you be doing the exam? I don't want you to get late."

At the end of my rotation, I saw, for the first time, a late-second-trimester aborted fetus. Its tiny, near-human limbs were what really got to me. It had its hand up near its mouth, as if to suck its miniature thumb. It was so delicate and vulnerable. Through the translucent skin, I could see highways of veins and arteries, little organs just germinating, little eyes that would never see. It was all wrapped in a plastic tissue disposal bag. My stomach churned. That night, I couldn't stop dreaming of babies calling out my name.

Motherhood, and therefore, pregnancy, has always been a cherished goal for me. My strong relationship with my own mother, as well as the central, almost divine, position that motherhood is given in my culture does not make me consider the matter lightly. When I watched the blood and tissue be removed from woman after woman, when I saw the little aborted fetus, my heart sank—because each was a loss. Not of life (for I cannot, do not believe that a fetus is an independent being, a life beyond the mother's body) but of potential—a potential child, a potential mother. But as my teary, motherly, premenopausal patient taught me, abortion is not the antithesis of motherhood. It is, instead, a way that motherhood is protected, and made a conscious, loving, and cognizant choice.

Abortion is never easy. Each of the many women's faces I saw, from an Eastern European immigrant, to a street-smart fourteen-year-old, to a premenopausal mother, were individuals with their own life stresses, their own reasons for deciding to get an abortion. I think of their many faces, and realize that abortion is so much more than a political belief, than a cause, than a slogan. While women's rights must be protected *en masse*, our dignity can only be protected one woman at a time.

Little White Pills

Science is great. All bow to the power of almighty science.

Old wives' tales, homeopathy, ayurveda, grandma's advice, lotions, potions, and old-time notions are all bunk. Junk. Throw them away, kerplunk.

But what if?

But when?

But I heard?

Like most of us, I grew up under the care of a family of non-doctors. Through childhood illnesses, bang-ups, cuts, and scrapes, as well as a host of exotic parasitic infestations (courtesy of summer vacations to Calcutta), I survived with a combination of allopathic (traditional, Western) medicine and homeopathy, potions, and lots of grandmotherly wisdom.

Common colds, headaches, and tummy upsets were first treated with my mother's mysterious arsenal: a box of little, white homeopathic pills imported from India. In addition to these sugary delights that my mother intermittently sprinkled under my upturned tongue, there was a host of grandmother-inspired complementary therapies. For the upset tummy, a bland meal of boiled rice, daal, and potatoes. For allergies, daily helpings of

91

bitter gourd. And my favorite, the nighttime treat for the common cold, was the "egg flip"—a frothy concoction of milk, honey, beaten egg, and the smallest smidgen of brandy. I've often suspected it was this last ingredient that was the real kicker, with the others thrown in to appease my mother's Victorian sensibilities lest she feel guilty about plying her ill child with the devil's brew.

Beyond this regimen, there were always the trips to my grandfather's favorite homeopath: an old buddy from the days of India's revolution. Every summer vacation in India, I would make a pilgrimage to the old doctor's chambers.

"What is your complaint?" he would intone blandly without looking up from his rickety desk. Little did I know, the question was not meant for me, but the adults in the room. Even as a teenager, it was clear that the homeopathic medical establishment expected me to be seen, and not heard.

But like the bullheaded American I was, I would respond. "I get a lot of sore throats," I remember saying once. "Whenever I'm tired, or out in the dust, or staying up too late. I thought you might be able to give me something to bolster my immune system."

"Tell your daughter," he intoned to my mother over his crooked wire-frame lenses, utterly ignoring me, "to take four drops of this." He scribbled on a sheet of paper, no prescription pad here. "In room-temperature water in the morning and in the evening. On an empty stomach, after rinsing her mouth out only. And not to eat anything for at least half an hour before or afterward. Also, don't store this near perfume, or spices, or anything with a strong scent."

Finally, he looked up at me, to utter briefly, "You obviously talk too much. Your personality is very energetic, hyper." Before I had a chance to protest, he added, "And you probably like to eat tart things." When my mother nodded affirmation, he looked down at his desk again, satisfied. "No tart things, and follow that prescription."

The entire interview, diagnosis, and treatment took about eight minutes.

But then, I never suffered from strep throat again.

This is but one example of such a homeopathic encounter, and I would never have even thought to mention it had I not encountered such blatant resistance to complimentary therapies in medical school. In my experience, traditional therapies are just like modern antibiotics—while they don't always work, they sometimes do. I still swear by one homeopathic concoction for my pollution and dust allergy. It's the best decongestant I've ever taken. A couple dashes of little white pills and my sinuses whoosh out a maelstrom. This effect, which I've found is hardly diminished by proximity to perfumes, spices, or non-empty stomachs, may seem like a bunch of hocus-pocus to most Westerners, but I don't think it's that different from most allopathic medical encounters.

For instance, in my teenage years, my allopathic doctor was a certain Dr. Patel, an Indian immigrant like my parents, who had a booming family practice near our New Jersey home. During my many bouts of wintertime sore throat, he would alleviate my suffering with a no-nonsense approach. "Take a needle," he would singsong in his heavily accented English while already in the process of swabbing my arm. "Needle will make you better."

While Dr. Patel's bedside manner (or lack of) might

not be the Western medicine norm, his perspective is perhaps a good representation of the Western medical philosophy. You patient, me doctor. Take needle, feel better.

From the less-than-medically-informed perspective, it often amounts to no more than hand waving. Take magic needle, feel better. Why? Because the doctor, like Simon, says so. Not much different than a demon-possessed tribal asking his priest to make a house call.

But, one might say, didn't you feel better? The answer, of course, is yes. Because even if Dr. Patel wasn't willing to explain, there was a very good rationale to his actions. Not magic, but an antibiotic. Not a demon, but a bacteria. Similarly, as research is beginning to prove, many homeopathic and other complimentary treatments also have sound scientific merit. And, like the headache commercial says, they work. Most importantly, unlike antibiotics and other allopathic treatments, they usually have minimal side effects.

But of course, you'll never catch those little white pills in the halls of Johns Hopkins.

Indeed, it was not until I came to medical school that I really realized the antagonism that exists between Western medicine and more traditional healing practices. "You won't believe the crap this family pulled off the Internet," I remember a resident once complaining, "and the patient's room is filled with a bunch of new-age guru books." He had snorted condescendingly, "Next thing you know they'll be asking me to light incense and chant mantras before every treatment!"

Then, perhaps remembering my ethnicity a little bit too late, he had muttered, "Oh, sorry. But you know what I mean."

I did know what he meant. And I can't help but snort in condescension myself. Because a few weeks after that very comment, a most difficult and interesting case presented itself to my friend Amy's medical team.

The patient was admitted sometime in the evening. Although Amy wasn't on call, she heard the story soon thereafter. It was a twenty-something-year-old young man who was in great agony from a non-life-threatening but utterly devastating phenomenon: continuous hiccups that had plagued him for the last four days. The patient and his wife were almost in tears. They had tried everything, from holding his breath, to scaring him, to turning upside down after gulping down tumblers of water. Commonsense cures had failed them. And so they turned to the great mecca of medical science for an answer.

"What about a sedative?" one resident had suggested.

"A neuroleptic?" another had asked.

As it turned out, the problem plagued the team for the greater part of twenty-four hours. In the meantime, the young patient was IV-ed, swathed in a hospital gown, and put on his insurance company's ticking bill. He lay inert in the country's bastion of medical research, the greatest minds of science turning cartwheels all around him.

The residents on call were apparently up much of the night doing extensive med-line searches on the issue.

"What's the latest, cutting-edge research that's out there?" they asked each other.

And the answer, in a burst of brilliance from the heavens, had come in the form of a research article in one of the world's leading medical journals. The powerful cure was not on the hospital formulary, in the crash carts, or on the shelves of the pharmacists. And so the two residents bustled down to the hospital cafeteria full of great import, and brought up the little, precious, paper-swathed panacea on a stolen hospital tray.

In a flash of light, to the symphony of a celestial choir, there it was. Pure, white, crystalline.

Sugar.

After a mouthful and a half, with the eyes of an advanced medical team upon him, the patient was cured.

I imagine he wept copiously, bowing before the healing hands that had fought and won against the demonic foe. Or perhaps he threw off his gown, cursed his insurance bill, and fumed at his wife for making him come to the hospital instead of just calling his Nana.

It just goes to show, whether antibiotic, homeopathy, or sugar, there's usually a little white pill appropriate for the situation. And rather than blindly believing in any one of them, or blindly disregarding any other, each should be taken in its own context, and measured for its own merit. For me, I take it all with a pinch of salt.

Or sometimes, something sweeter.

Revelations

During the bubonic plague, physicians who cared for the sick wore complicated paraphernalia, including beaklike hoods that made them look like malevolent birds, to protect themselves from infection. Regardless of these precautions, history tells us that doctors of plague victims were treated with as much fear and loathing as the disease itself, as if, in their ornithological costumes, they personified the bird of death.

I grew up in the era of a modern plague, and by the time I was applying to medical school, I had to confront a social anxiety that disfigured the medical profession as much as any beaklike hood. My family worried about my risks of HIV infection on the job, and even I grew concerned as some of my pre-med friends opted not to apply to medical school because of HIV. Health care reform was decreasing medical salaries, certain professions were overrun with physicians, and now, doctors were at risk of a deadly infection. It was the early 1990s, and people were afraid.

Although research on HIV and AIDS influenced a significant portion of my basic science education, it was not until the beginning of clinical rotations that my medical school class was seriously taught universal precautions. That was when the risk of acquiring HIV infection as a student really hit home. I was paranoid the first time I had to draw blood, and fumbled awkwardly, causing the patient to cry out in pain. It's not easy to do a venipuncture when you're trying not to use your fingers.

I never directly took care of a patient with HIV, however, until my internal medicine rotation. It was a typical, prolonged call night, and I was waiting around to pick up a new patient. The few who came in at a reasonable hour were deemed too "ordinary" by my intern, who, like a typical resident, told me, "Those patients aren't interesting enough. Why don't you wait around for a zebra?" The thought was that real physicians passed up plain old horses for their striped, exotic, rarer cousins. But the evening grew longer with absolutely no signs of Serengeti wildlife.

I was hovering around the nurses' station, hoping for a patient, when I heard that there was a new occupant in room 30. My intern was down in the Emergency Room, so like any eager med student, I headed off to interview my new patient. Maybe I would get home before 3 A.M. after all.

It was the last room at the end of the hallway, the one next to the abandoned nursing station. It was so dark and quiet that I initially doubted there was anyone in there. Then I saw a young African American man sitting quietly on the edge of the bed with only the dim bedside light illuminating his gaunt face. His hollow cheeks emphasized the roundness of his red-rimmed eyes, while drawing his face into an angular point. His clothes were tattered, dirty, and less-than-pleasant smelling. In fact, the entire room reeked of sweat and decay. The young man was studying his blackened, cracked nails, and looked up cautiously when I walked in. He eyed me, a small Indian American woman whose white coat, beeper, and clipboard belied her unsure step. He stared, saying nothing.

"Mr., umm," I looked down surreptitiously at my clipboard, "Martin, I'm the student doctor on the team, and . . ."

Mr. Martin, like most patients, looked a little skeptical at my identity as a "student doctor." What exactly did that mean? his face seemed to ask. I wasn't sure I knew myself.

As I continued my stilted, medical student–style interview, it became clear that Mr. Martin was neither eager to listen nor participate. Finally, I stopped the barrage of memorized queries, and asked, "Mr. Martin, why are you here?"

His voice was a little gravelly, but clear. It was a lot younger than he looked. "Rob," he said, "my name's Rob."

Feeling more than a bit ridiculous, I discarded my unnaturally stiff attitude, the "professional distance" I had been taught to always observe. I decided to begin again. "Hi, Rob," I said, extending my hand, "I'm Sayantani."

After that, it was much easier. I perched myself up on the windowsill to hear his story.

"I'm twenty years old," he told me, and I tried to hide my surprise. He was five years younger than I was at the time, but looked at least ten years older. He didn't seem to notice, continuing, "I ain't been feelin' too good lately. I'm supposed to be livin' with my aunt, but I been livin' in between friends' houses for a couplea weeks now, and the last couplea days on the street. I been partyin' a lot lately."

When I probed a little further, I realized that for Rob, "partying" meant IV heroin, and sharing needles. I asked him in what way he wasn't feeling well, and he told me, "I been losin' weight, I ain't been hungry, and yesterday, I fainted. I didn't wanna, but my lady friend made me come in."

As he spoke, his voice became coarser and coarser. His story ended in a torrent of coughing. I handed him a cup, and tried not to appear startled at the blood-tinged sputum he produced.

Finally, I came to the part of the interview where I had to ask the question of questions. "Have you ever been tested for HIV?"

When he replied negatively, I continued, "Does anyone in your life have HIV or AIDS?"

Rob paused for a minute, looking down at his nails for an answer. Then, without much emotion, he said, "My dad died from AIDS when I was fourteen."

I murmured my sympathies. He added, "We used to party together. He's the one who taught me how to shoot up."

There was pin-drop silence. Rob's coarse breathing seemed very loud in my ears, his smell overwhelmingly pungent. I wished I hadn't turned on the fluorescent lights, which made the room appear even more stark and impersonal. I fidgeted for a moment on my windowsill perch, looking down at the chic new shoes my mother had bought me on my last trip home. Suddenly, achingly, the memory of that shoe-shopping trip popped into my mind. The shiny, artificial environment of the mall, the soothing smell of leather, the obsequious salesman who had waited on us seemed both longingly familiar and an eternity away. I wanted that security again. This world of

Rob's, of the hospital, of medicine was too frightening for a little Indian woman from the New Jersey 'burbs. I fought an overwhelming urge to bolt out of the room.

But instead of running away, I did what logically came next, a physical exam. From head to toe, as I had been taught, checking off system by system, I examined my new patient. It didn't take me long to make a presumptive diagnosis. The warm, sallow skin on his face was checkered with distinctive discolorations I had long ago learned to name; his foul-smelling mouth housed not only decaying teeth and gums, but a frothy white blanket over cheek and tongue. They were Kaposi's sarcoma and thrush—two telltale signs of immunocompromise. Rob probably had AIDS.

My initial reaction to these discoveries would only a moment later disgust me. For instead of feeling sorrow, or empathy, I felt a distinctive surge of elation. I had what every medical student wanted: an answer. I would not be humiliated at morning rounds, I would not be pummeled with confusing, unanswerable questions. I had done what every med student longed to do: I had made a new diagnosis.

It is a bitter experience to elate at another's misfortune. I couldn't believe that I had done it. Yet, the fact was, I knew I would be rewarded for Rob's terrible tragedy. My team would say that I had "hopped on the new AIDS guy," that I had "bulldogged the case." They would pump up my ego by telling me I had done "strong work." For once, I would not feel stupid, or useless, or inferior. For once, I would not feel tears rising unbidden to my eyes in the hospital.

On that last point, however, I was wrong. It was not my

team, but Rob himself who made me cry that night. Unaware of the emotions surging around in me, he asked me a serious, trusting question.

"Doc, am I goin' to be all right?" His voice was quiet.

It was the "doc" that really got to me. Rob's eyes, which had been at first so cautious of me, were suddenly full of trust. I babbled nervously about having to speak to my team, about having to do tests. I don't think I fooled him.

"Can you call my aunt?" he asked next, his voice tremulous. "I'd like to see my aunt. She's gonna be worryin' about me. I didn't want to worry her."

I took his aunt's number and promised to call in the morning. It was getting late, and the nurses were busily weighing, undressing, and IV-ing Rob. I gathered my papers together, and bid him goodnight.

I presented my formal history and physical to my team in the morning, who popped cursorily in Rob's room to confirm my physical findings. The Kaposi's and the thrush were unmistakable, and after we left the room, just as I had suspected, I was given accolades. "She had worked him up before I even had a look at him," my intern boasted.

"Good job," said the attending physician vaguely in my direction. "Just make sure you go and tell him his diagnosis as soon as the CD4 count comes in."

"Don't you wait for the HIV test to come up positive?" I asked.

"For a definite diagnosis, sure," the attending agreed, "but in this case, a low T cell count is good enough. We have to let him know what we think it is." The physician looked at me directly. "This is your patient now, so make sure you prepare him for his prognosis."

I suppose he meant to make me feel proud, honored. Yet the burden of having Rob Martin be considered my patient alone and the responsibility of having to give him a presumptive AIDS diagnosis even before the HIV test results were in was overwhelming. Even after Rob's CD4 came back ridiculously low, I was too intimidated by the hierarchy of medicine to ask for assistance or guidance in how to break the news to him. So I did the best that I could. I wish now I had done more.

He was dozing in bed but looked up expectantly when I walked in. "Did you call my aunt?" he asked worriedly.

I nodded briefly, omitting the fact that his aunt had repeatedly demanded to know if her nephew had "the AIDS." "I knew he was sick," she said. "I knew he'd get 'the AIDS,' just like his daddy. I told that boy, I told him." Then the woman had become hysterical. "Doc, you gotta look after my boy. Tell him I'm gonna try to come see him today, but I don't know. There's a lotta buses you gotta take all the way across town to the hospital. I don't know if I'm gonna make it. But you let him know I'm gonna try. You hear? You let him know I'm gonna try." A pause. "But it shore is a lotta buses."

I hadn't revealed anything to the aunt, grateful that the strict rules of patient confidentiality prevented me from saying much except that her nephew was in our care. I wished my team had given me some sort of similar guideline as to what they expected me to tell Rob now that his CD4 count was 63.

I perched up on my windowsill again and glanced at Rob's anxious face. He knew I had something to tell him. In the daylight, he now looked younger than his twenty years. Cleaned up, clothed in a blue hospital gown, he looked strangely fragile, like some gaunt, gawky bird whose elegance was in his very awkwardness. He played with his thickened, black thumbnail while he waited for me to speak.

"Rob," my voice sounded thready. I cleared my throat, and willed my voice to go down an octave. "Rob," I began again, "I've got something important to talk about. Your HIV test isn't back yet, but another test which measures your white blood cells, your CD4 cells, has come back very low."

"What d'ya mean?" He stared at me steadily.

"Well, there's a few things this could mean, but the thing all the doctors here are worried about is AIDS." I didn't know how else to say it. He must suspect, I told myself, it can't be a surprise.

It was. Rob's dark face went ashen and he started halfway up, but then fell back against the pillows, a sickened look on his face. Then, without preface, his face split with a squawking wail. I was stunned. "We won't know anything for sure until we have the HIV test back," I stammered. "I just wanted you to know what the possibility was."

He wasn't listening to me. He was wailing. At first, it was just sounds—birdlike, animal-like. He was a tortured creature caught in a hunter's snare. Then, he called to me. "Doc!" he wailed. "Doc! What am I gonna do? What am I gonna do, Doc?"

"You're going to wait until the test results come in for sure," I reemphasized, my stomach a churning knot. Why hadn't I waited? Why hadn't I asked for help? There were properly trained HIV counselors in the hospital, why hadn't I called one of them? Why had my team sent me in here to do this terrible task with no preparation? How had they thought I was prepared for this? How had I?

"I'm scared, Doc!" he choked out, then suddenly quieted. His face searched mine. "I'm really scared."

I moved over to the bed, picking up his rough, dry hand in my own. "I know," I said, my own voice shaky. "I know."

"I'm scared, I'm scared," he kept repeating over and over, leaning forward to rest on my shoulder. I patted him awkwardly, terrified at what I had done, terrified for what lay in store for him. He called me "Doc," yet I felt as competent as a child. I had been sent to do an onerous task with no warning of the gravity it held. Because of my own naiveté, I had put Rob through a difficult situation. I had very few answers for him. The only thing I could give him was comfort.

I sat with him for a while, until he had recovered his composure. I had made a move to go at that point, but he stopped me. "Stay a little?" he had asked. And so I sat with Rob, chatting about the latest movies, our favorite superstars, our favorite musicians. We talked about his father. We talked about how to tell his aunt of his potential condition. When his voice grew strained from all the crying and talking, I left to let him sleep.

Outside Rob's room, I let myself feel the impact of what I had done. I felt shocked, and bruised, and humbled. I wasn't sure if I had made a grave mistake, though I was sure that my intentions had been honorable. It was glamorous to think of myself as the one person who had at least taken the time to care for Rob—his angel of mercy. Yet I was not sure I was anything but an ill-advised student who had abused a patient's emotions due to her own lack of training. Far from an angel, I was perhaps for Rob the beak-hooded symbol of death that physicians had been during that earlier plague.

I looked down at the shoes my mother had bought me and wished I could click them three times together. Perhaps they would grow wings and carry me to some safe and secure place. I wished with all my might to fly home.

Darth Vader Hoods
and Bunny Suits

A not so long time ago, in a galaxy quite close by, there was a young rebel fighting an educational battle with an empirelike institution. Like a laser-spewing Death Star, the Empire bombarded her with information and facts and she fought her way bumblingly through their onslaught. Her faulty memory was a mediocre light saber, but she charged on, hoping against hope that the Force would, for once, be with her.

The first time I saw *Star Wars*, I was too young to read the scrolling words on the screen at the beginning of the movie. Regardless, George Lucas's epic fable had a great impact upon me, as it did most young people of my generation. I spent many Halloweens with symmetrical croissantlike hairpieces pinned to my head. Beyond the obvious attraction of Princess Leia's bouffant, the film taught me about honor, valor, and courage against all odds. The indomitable Princess, the first adventure heroine I had ever seen on screen, was a role model of female verve and uppityness. I dreamed of growing up to defend my galaxy against the Dark Side.

Twenty years after I first saw *Star Wars*, the epic trilogy was again packing American movie theaters. My overactive six-year-old imagination could hardly have predicted where twenty years would bring me. At twenty-six, I was not only able to follow Lucas's scrolling cinematic introduction, but I was well on my way to becoming a physician/rebel. The medical school experience, has, however, oftentimes been a struggle between forces light and dark. Nowhere was this perhaps more true than during my third-year surgery rotation.

Surgery, with its elaborate costumes and theatrical operating stage, is nothing short of cinematic material. To its credit, it affords students a rare opportunity to peek into the awe-inspiring galaxies of human anatomy; to tinker, if you will, with the internal universe. However, surgery as a required third-year medical student rotation inspires dread of mythic proportions. Five-thirty A.M. morning rounds, every third night overnight "call," and endless hours of mindless clamp holding punctuated only by unexpected and esoteric questioning ("pimping") by arrogant surgeon-teachers inspires terror in all but a few medical students. Needless to say, I was dreading surgery.

The first thing that students must learn during their surgical rotation is the elaborate process of scrubbing in. What may, to novices, look like nothing more than washing one's hands is in fact a highly ritualistic ceremony denoting hierarchy and tradition. It is the transition from the world of the "unscrubbed" to the "scrubbed"— the, if you will, darkness to the light. Unlike in the movies, however, there is seldom much guidance given to novices regarding the ritual of scrubbing; no Yoda to teach young medical knights. The first time I scrubbed in, I clumsily bumbled my way through the procedure, frightened that I would be scolded for "breaking scrub"— that is, touching my sterile hands or forearms to anything nonsterile, such as my chest, sides, another surgeon's back, nondraped tables, etc. Elbows aloft off chest, hands in air, my nose itching desperately beneath my surgical mask, I was being taught to respect the medical Force.

Like the ever-present white robes of Luke and Leia, surgical scrubbing has its own costuming as well. From the slippery paper bootie (which never seems to quite protect my sneakers from stains), to the hat-head-inducing surgical cap, to the masks which, once put on, immediately seem to cause one's nose to run profusely. Fearful of untoward splashes reaching my eyes, I usually chose a mask with an attached Storm Trooper–like vertical plastic eye shield. The critical trick to this mask is to pinch it tightly at the nose—otherwise the vapor of one's own breath inevitably steams up the inside of the eye shield. The first time I wore one, I had to suffer blindly through the haze during a long surgery. I actually made myself dizzy because I started breathing shallowly to try and prevent the rolling clouds of fog in front of my eyes. I doubt Lucas's Imperial Storm Troopers had similar problems.

These are the basics, the standard backdrop to every cinematic surgical performance. The scene opens with the pushing open of the O.R. door with one's behind, and backing into the brightly lit equipment-filled stage. After this point, there are specific nuances to each and every type of surgical show. I realized this during my orthopedic surgery rotation. Orthopedic surgeons, who hammer, chisel, and drill arms, legs, and various joints back into proper working order, are not an innately theatrical bunch. They are what is derogatorily known as "orthopods" or "bone docs"—the supposed jocks of the surgical world.

Despite any lack of inherent artistic sensibility, an orthopedic surgery is quite a dramatic spectacle to watch, made more so by the theatrical array of surgical gear. The most striking of these costumes is the Darth Vader surgical hood, part of the airtight space suit–like costumes that surgeons wear during large joint operations to protect patients from infection. The first total hip replacement I attended, I feared toppling over from the awkwardness of the surgical gear. The air rushing around within my hood made an ominous "whooshing" that I could only liken to Lord Vader's raspy breath. I wondered if I, like Luke's father, had become trapped within the Dark Lord's body.

"Suction!" the attending surgeon must have said, but I could only see her mouth move. My head was heavy with a whooshing hurricane. I stared at her, flabbergasted, only figuring out what I was supposed to do by the frantic hand gestures of one of the residents. I suppose the swirls of oozing blood obscuring her surgical field clued me in as well. It's hard to look smart with Darth Vader breathing heavy in your ears.

Costuming difficulties are not confined to orthopedic surgery. My favorite cocktail party story actually involves a general surgery mishap. The cast of characters is an emergency late night surgery, a naughty scrub machine, and an Imperial attending surgeon who puts George Lucas's wickedly wizened Emperor to shame.

The scene opens as follows: It is after midnight on the general surgery service when a call is received concerning a tragic auto accident and an emergency surgery admission. The case is complicated, and the attending surgeon on call is summoned in. As it happens, this fateful night of all nights, the very chief of surgery himself is on call. He is an elderly British man, rigorously trained at the Royal College of Surgeons in not only surgical technique, but gentlemanly behavior and physician etiquette. His carriage is regally upright, evidence of his military past. During surgeries, he speaks poetically about his time in the Boer Wars, and every resident nods thoughtfully. "Yes, my boys!" he booms majestically (he is from a time when ladies did not enter fields of battle or surgery, and he cannot bring himself to recognize the surgical presence of the fairer sex), "to become a great surgeon, you must first be a great man!" The residents, rolling their eyes, drone, "Yes, sir." An Emperor, after all, cannot be contradicted.

That night, in the operating room, the forces of light and dark compete head to head. A vascular surgeon and orthopedic surgeon work on different body parts of the injured patient while the general surgery residents prepare for the arrival of their Imperial leader. There is no room at the operating table for assistants, students, or nurses. A surgeon barks for an instrument. The nurse bumps someone's arm in the process of handing it over and breaks her own and the other person's scrub. The instruments clatter to the floor. Tensions run high. For a moment, the patient's vital signs destabilize. If you listen hard, you can hear the goose-stepping clatter of Imperial Storm Troopers approaching. The music plays ominously.

The Emperor's shuttlecraft has landed, and he is en route to the battlefield. On the way, he must stop for a change of Imperial costume. He punches his size, extra-large, into the automated scrub-dispensing machine. At this witching hour, the laundry services have fallen behind. The machine is out of extra-large scrubs. The Emperor re-punches another code. The machine is out of large scrubs as well. He contemplates for a moment, but soon rejects the idea of stuffing his regal body into medium scrubs. The troops must not see their leader popping out of a too-tight uniform. It wouldn't do to break the young men's morale.

The Emperor, a resourceful man who has seen more than one battle in his time (has he told you about the time he was in the Boer Wars?) has an idea. He will don the common garb of electricians, construction men, and pharmacy representatives when they enter the holy regions of the "scrubbed." It is a costume nicknamed the Bunny Suit—a yellow, papery, foot-to-neck zip-up oversuit. It would have normally been beneath a man of the Emperor's standing to wear such clothes, but in a time of crisis, a leader has to bend. His men need him.

The scene switches to the operating room again. The music swells to mark the rising tension. The Emperor has not arrived, and the troops are getting edgy. The life force is ebbing out of their patient. The tension in the room is at an all-time peak. The residents wield their light saber–like scalpels without much confidence. They need their leader to guide them. But then, the music changes, indicating the arrival of the Emperor. The troops are at attention. Everyone looks expectantly at the door.

The door swings open from a confident push. A man strides into the brightly lit room, bristling with regal authority. "Well, boys, what do you have there?" he booms. No one answers. The man growls, impatient. "Gentlemen! When I ask a question, I expect an answer!"

The room is still with pin-drop silence. In the fluorescent overhead lights, the leader is revealing more than he intended. His paper-thin Bunny Suit, zipped on over nothing but pale flesh and white cotton briefs, is hardly regal covering. Indeed, under the bright operating-room lights, it is clear to everyone that the Emperor isn't wearing clothes.

For a moment he stares indignantly back at a roomful of shocked faces. Then, looking down on himself, the Emperor lets out a soldierlike curse. "These bloody things are see-through, aren't they?" he bellows as he scurries out of the room.

The Imperial troops haven't had a laugh like that in ages. They howl hysterically beneath their masks, careful not to wipe their streaming eyes so as not to break scrub. Whether or not the Force was with them, at least for once, they have had a great chuckle.

If I Had a Hammer (would that make me more of a woman?)

"Do you want to hold it?"

It was a provocative question.

I hesitated for a minute. I had never held something that powerful in my hands. "Umm . . . OK," I answered after a brief spasm of fear.

And then there it was. Vibrating. In my hands. The power, the majesty, the awesomeness of it: the most enormous drill I had ever seen in my life. And I had it in my hands. More than that, I was operating it. I was controlling it. And I was using it to set a new hip on a woman who might otherwise have never walked again.

The orthopedic surgeon standing next to me had her hands a few inches away from mine the whole time, but I was the one in charge. It was a heady, almost drunken feeling of power. I was not only drilling a woman's hip all by myself, but I was doing it right.

"Good job," the doctor said briefly when the case was finished. It was extravagant praise for me. I beamed under my mask, and almost floated out of the O.R. I felt, for the first time in medical school, macho.

Man and machine. Woman and nature. The dichotomy is an old one. We of the "weaker sex" don't change our own oil, we don't operate cranes, and we definitely don't

drill. Or at least, that's the idea. And the schism is obviously deeply socialized. Otherwise, why would a
brief episode as a "toolwoman" make me, a person who
prides herself on her gender politics, feel so imbued
with machismo?

When I was a little girl, I wasn't exactly a mechanical
whiz. Consistent with gender stereotypes, I enjoyed
playing with my Barbies over doing anything vaguely
mechanical. My father, a mechanical engineer, wanted
his only child to excel at the hard sciences, and tried
desperately to improve my visual-spatial abilities with
puzzles, logical games, and, when I was about eleven
years old, an Erector Set. (Pretty Freudian name for a
construction set, which was surely designed with little
prepubescent boys in mind. Of course, as a profound line
from a silly movie says, "Freud didn't know dick about
women.") When I exhibited less than profound enthusiasm for the toy, my father did a less than feminist thing.
He teased me about my lack of spatial skills, and allowed
me to stuff the entire kit into a dark corner of my closet.
(He's been a wonderful father, but assuredly, that wasn't
his strongest moment.)

And so, I grew up avoiding to my utmost anything
mechanical beyond programming a VCR. I convinced
myself that I was so terrible at visual-spatial things that I
wouldn't even hammer a nail if I could avoid it. When I
was handed that orthopedic drill, it was more than the
fear of a new surgical procedure that made my stomach
drop to the floor. The woman orthopedic surgeon who
handed me that loudly buzzing instrument, a rare breed
in and of herself, made me do an even rarer thing. She
made me confront my own fear of the mechanical and
win. Although she surely didn't realize the depth of my

fear of machines, I will always be grateful to her just for
that opportunity.

Orthopedic surgery wasn't the first time I had to confront that enormous a medical instrument. During Gross
Anatomy, there was a big buzz saw we used to drill into
the cadaver's skull. It was plugged into an outlet in the
ceiling, and hung down from a thick cord like some horrible metal phallic thing. We used it near the end of dissection class, which is good, because we medical students
were fairly desensitized to all things gross by that point.
But even then, drilling day wasn't pretty. The process
made an awful burning smell and caused chips of bone to
fly everywhere. When one of the students at the next
table used it, it actually flew, lifelike, out of his hands and
proceeded to jump around his dissection table like some
monstrous creature escaped from a choke collar. It
didn't cause much havoc only because its wild leaping
caused it to unplug itself. It sure did scare the hell out of
everyone, though. After seeing that, I wasn't brave
enough to wield the saw even once. My all-women team
of dissectors played rock, paper, scissors until one of us
was unlucky enough to get voted into the inauspicious
office.

But all of that changed with my orthopedic surgery
course. I only rotated on the service for two weeks. And
of that time, operated with the female attending of the
medical drill incident only twice. It wasn't as if we had
the time to form anything more than a strictly professional relationship. In fact, she wasn't even that great of a
conversationalist. I remember gaping moments of silence during our one-on-one daily lectures. She would
talk, off the top of her head, about orthopedic topics of
interest, and then ask me a number of questions. It was

the same old pimping that I dreaded. And yet, there was something different, too. Even though I got very few of the answers right at first, she did not change her attitude toward me at all. No scolding, no scorn, not even the slightest tone of condemnation. She maintained her professional, crisp attitude and did something few other attendings would ever do. She would tell me the right answer to every single question I got wrong, adding a few other relevant tidbits. When she asked me about the same subject again, it was easy for me to answer correctly because it had been explained to me. I never felt stupid. I was motivated to study and impress my attending. And most importantly, I learned.

She was an odd, abrupt person. But funny, too. She would crack jokes with her dry sense of humor that usually took me about a minute to understand. She knew, for instance, that the rest of the team, the male residents, detested and feared her. In fact, they told me horror stories about her that weren't at all consistent with my experience. They called her "the dragon."

"Those little arrogant pricks deserve to be afraid of somebody." She laughed lightly, and smiled at me with something resembling indulgence. In retrospect, it was probably one of the only times in medical school I saw the Old Girl network in operation.

There were pictures of her, quite dashing in flight gear, decorating the walls of her office. With her short hair, reflective glasses, and tall stature, she didn't look very different from the all-male helicopter crew around her. She was a woman, a physician, and an orthopedic surgeon in this man's army. Each of the three were rarities in that environment, and each required, as she explained to me, that she prove herself over and over.

She wasn't exactly a revolutionary, though. "They had to respect a woman who could drink them under the table," she once said blandly.

I only guessed that this physician was, in addition, something else that the military does not respond well to: a lesbian. Like the armed forces, I did not ask, and was not told. But in her office, during our lecture sessions, I felt a bond between us formed from the knowledge that she, too, was a vulnerable person in the complicated, often oppressive world of medicine. And that in her strange, silent way, she was looking out for me.

There are few out gay men, lesbians, or bisexuals at Hopkins. That's not to say they aren't there. It's just that the conservative environment doesn't exactly encourage a spectrum of sexualities. As a woman who dates men, I guess I don't have a right to say what Hopkins is like for gays and lesbians. But I do know that there were no out gay people in my class. I also know that the few people who were out to me ended up, by the end of medical school, dating people of the opposite gender. I'm not suggesting that those straight relationships weren't valid, or real, or loving. It is just disturbing that people who previously had same-sex relationships, and had to some extent recognized and celebrated their gay identities, somehow felt that they had to not only hide this part of themselves during medical school, but express their sexuality only via heterosexual means.

The homophobic environment of Hopkins is perfectly exemplified by a comment made to me by a classmate when she learned the identity of my orthopedic surgery attending. "Oh, her," she said demeaningly. "God, there aren't anything but butches in ortho, are there?"

I protested her use of the pejorative, and she apologized. But it was enough to remind me what medical training might have been like for my newest physician-teacher.

I don't think I realized the depth of my ortho attending's support even during my rotation; it was months later, when I read my clinical evaluation. Before that point, most of my evaluations said that I was "a team player," "a joy to work with," "cooperative," "enthusiastic," and "diligent." Female qualities, if ever I heard them. My orthopedic surgery grade was not only an A++, the highest I got throughout medical school, but the accompanying handwritten evaluation said that I had "great surgical hands," that I was "a prize assistant surgeon," and that I would do well in "any of the surgical specialties." It was the most flattering, empowering, macho thing I have ever read about myself. And when I did, I did quite a stereotypically feminine thing. I cried.

It's not that one simple incident with an orthopedic tool had made me into some mechanical genius. But rather, that a woman I hardly knew, a woman who could have, like so many others, made me feel bad about myself, instead made me feel wonderful, if only for a moment. The weird thing is, that wonderfulness was somehow born of, not human contact (because we heard more silence than speech) but of a machine. For that brief instant when she let me wield that enormous drill, she made me feel something I rarely felt during my medical education: that I could be a doctor.

It's of course ironic, based on my opinions of the military, that it should be an air force orthopedic surgeon who was the closest thing to a mentor I ever had during a medical rotation. Of course, that mentorship came less from our interactions than from my own ideas about her.

She never told me much about herself, never asked me much about myself, and definitely never laughed with me, cried with me, or came close to hugging me. If it wasn't for those glimpses of the Old Girl network she showed me, I might have even thought that she was nothing more than another woman who accepted and excelled at the masculine medical culture. But instead of boxing me out, she drilled a tiny hole, almost imperceptible, into the traditional medical armor. She made a tiny space for me to see the light.

If I had a hammer, (or a drill, or a buzz saw, or some power), I'd try to use that tool wisely to, like that flight-doc orthopod, hammer out spaces for the women who came after me.

The question that remains, however, is whether I really want a hammer at all. To paraphrase Audre Lorde, if the master's tools can never be used to pull down the master's house, can the hammer of traditional medicine be used to reshape medical school?

Backside Barbers

A poker face is one of the primary assets in surgery. A field in which the main, and often only, questions asked to patients on morning rounds are, "Did you have a bowel movement?" and "Did you pass gas?" requires of its practitioners enormous solemnity and inner strength. For instance, a particularly hearing-impaired patient once needed my entire team of surgeons to shout, "Did you fart?" before he could manage a reply. When it was affirmative, the team all but did a jig.

A casual observer might think that the poker face is less of a critical requirement during the actual procedure of surgery, when the majority of one's face is covered by hat and mask. However, as anyone who has felt the urge to laugh during a complicated surgery will know, it's all in the eyes. More often than not, however, it was not laughter, but anger that I had to mask from my eyes during my third-year surgical rotation, since surgical humor is at best offensive. Men with hundred-thousand-dollar educations, worldwide credentials, and gifted talent share with each other jokes about bodily functions, sexual organs, and more often than not, women. The most popular surgical witticisms usually involve, in some way, shape, or form, Red Riding Hood, a blind priest, or three men of the cloth in a brothel. Highbrow humor, it is not. During such humorous and/or offensive moments, my poker face/eyes would be tested to their maximum, and so I would use the old Brady Bunch trick, imagining the surgeon stripped down to his unsterile undies in front of the entire operating team. When that didn't work, I just bit my lip until I drew blood.

The experience that most taxed my poker face during my surgical rotation, however, was not in the operating room or even on morning rounds. It was in surgery outpatient clinic. I had just made my way down to the outpatient department one Friday afternoon, prepared for a relatively relaxing few hours. Clinic, while the least favorite experience for most why-isn't-the-patient-knocked-out-yet-what-do-you-mean-I-have-to-talk-to-them surgery residents, was quite pleasurable for me as a third-year medical student. It was one of the few times I got to actually do something, instead of just holding, pulling, or suctioning. During clinic, the nonsurgically inclined med student can relax, removing staples and stitches, cleaning and packing abscesses, and even placing casts. Those few Friday afternoons were the times I actually got to practice my favorite part of medicine—talking to people about their lives, their problems, their stories. However, this particular Friday, I would face my greatest challenge in self control. I had to fight a quickly losing battle with my own sense of the hysterical.

I had just finished removing a young boy's stitches without making him yell, and was feeling rather proud of myself when the chief of surgery, a rather self-important British gentleman, beckoned me. "You, there, my girl, come, come quickly!" He gestured importantly even as I felt a pit of dread growing in my stomach. Surely he was about to ask me some obscure question that I would not be able to answer. "A very interesting case, yes, indeed, a very interesting case in Exam Room Two and Dr. Sweeney is in grave need of your assistance."

I felt relieved that he did not mean to immediately "pimp" me, but I was a little confused as to what assistance my surgical intern, David Sweeney, could "gravely" require from me. I regretted being paired up with him for what must be a fairly complicated and serious procedure. An attractive man who knew a little too well how good he looked, David had made me uncomfortable on more than one call night with his heavy-handed flirtation and intimate behavior. One night at 3 A.M. he had actually gotten down on his knees and mockingly proposed marriage to me in the physicians' lounge while I blushed, fidgeted, and wished I was anywhere but there. Even though I had tried to avoid sharing call nights with him after that, it seemed beyond my power. In short, he was making my rotation slightly hellish; but since he was in a position of relative authority over me, I didn't feel I could properly tell him off. It was no Clarence Thomas incident, yet it was making me awkward and uncomfortable. So, that afternoon, I had no desire to walk into the exam room with David—but I had to. With as little temerity as possible, I answered, "Yes, sir," and bowled into Examination Room 2.

The sight I saw upon opening that door will probably never be erased from my mind. David's face, usually cockily self-confident, or at least coyly flirtatious, bore an unrecognizable expression I could only liken to deep and utter pain. When I focused on what he was doing, I quickly knew why. Before David were the upturned round hills of a young woman's sizable buttocks, and the young doctor stood before this sight with glassy eyes and a tentatively held disposable shaving razor.

"Come, come, why the hesitation, Doctor?" The chief of surgery had walked into the tiny room on my heels. "With a pilonidal cyst, one must shave away any naughty hair growth! It is essential to remove each and every hair! Chop, chop, Doctor, get to it!" The Chief waved his arms in a flourish. "I have even brought you a lovely young assistant!"

While I would have normally taken umbrage to being called a "lovely young assistant," there was something humorous in imagining myself a sequin-clad assistant to David's mustachioed and caped magician. Indeed, Dr. Sweeney looked as if he wished his razor were a wand, and he could zap himself anyplace but where he was. He managed a wan smile to the departing chief of surgery, and then turned his harassed eyes to me. "Ahem," he began, clearing his throat. "This is Miss Jackson, and we're cleaning up the cyst in between her buttocks."

Miss Jackson, remarkably poised for a young woman in her undignified position, grinned cheerfully at me. "How ya doin'?" she chirped. I returned a friendly "hi."

"I'm having a bit of a hard time holding back her buttocks while I shave, so how about you stand here," David indicated the spot right in front of him, "and hold while I get all the hairs?"

"And I sure got a lot of 'em!" interjected the prone Miss Jackson. "I got so many hairs on my butt, I don't even know how they all got there!" A plethora of black and brown braids, which seemed an extension of Miss Jackson's quirky personality, bobbed pleasantly on her head while she talked. She lay calmly on her stomach, leaning slightly up on her elbows so that she could turn around and speak to us. Her demeanor, which was more like that of a woman suntanning on the beach than a patient in an embarrassing situation, made David look even more ridiculous.

The corners of my mouth quivered from the struggle of not smiling. It was an enormous pleasure to see the egotistical and overly self-confident David in a bind. Miss Jackson, with her cheerful disposition and chatty quips, was doing nothing for his image as an important physician being trained to save lives. I wondered if Miss Jackson realized the effect she was having on him. I felt like she was an extension of my ego, an absurd revenge created by my overactive imagination.

I turned to David with a pleasant smile. "Since you're stronger than me," I said, my eyes wide with innocence, "why don't *you* hold and *I* shave those naughty hairs?"

And so I spent the next twenty minutes dulling three razors on Miss Jackson's plentiful backside hair. I chatted pleasantly with my unwitting coconspirator, who informed me that she felt much more comfortable coming to the surgical clinic for the procedure than asking some member of her own family. I encouraged her to return to Dr. Sweeney again. He glared helplessly at me, his arms struggling in their attempt to part Miss Jackson's curvaceous backside. My vengeance tasted very sweet.

David couldn't look in my direction during the rest of the day. I was so hysterical in my triumph, it was all I could do not to laugh out loud. Even if I had donned a surgical mask to hide my grin, my eyes couldn't have stopped twinkling.

The Demons

Demons come in all shapes and sizes, but one thing is certain, they are sneaky little devils. They burrow into your skin when you least expect them, leaping out from behind giant shadows in your subconscious. During my fourth-year child and adolescent psychiatry elective, I realized much about both my young patients' and my own demons. Terrors are not restricted to the psychiatrically ill, I realized, nor are they limited to the workings of a murky mind. Rather, demons come in both internal and external varieties, and each is usually impacted by the other. Indeed, when I was a little brown girl growing up in the heart of the American Midwest, my most pesky external demons manifested themselves in my internal psyche. However, for a young patient whom I met during my rotation, internal demons took very real form in the external world.

"Don't laugh at me?" asks the little girl in a low voice, her eyes fixed, staring on an unidentifiable point in the floor.

"Of course not," I reassure her in my most even tones. "I'm here to listen, Alison; no one is going to laugh at

you." I glance at my attending physician, who nods reassuringly at us both.

As a child, my demons hid in most public places, laughing and giggling at me. I could not walk into a public restaurant with my oh-so-obviously-foreign family without feeling a thousand eyes upon me. My father was short and dark when others were tall and golden; my mother wore saris and went to grad school while others wore aprons and went to PTA meetings. I felt strangers' stares a thousandfold more intensely than my adult parents did. I could not walk into a public place without wanting the floor to open up and swallow me out of my misery.

"Don't laugh at me, OK?" Alison asks again, her voice shrill and brittle. "I'm asking you not to laugh at anything I might have to say. Don't any of you think I'm weird or anything." She lifts her tousled head and focuses wide, almost frenzied eyes on me. They are much older than Alison's twelve years. "Don't think I'm weird or anything," she repeats in a near murmur, swallowing her words into her secret turmoil.

The playground was particularly tough. At an age where it was critical to fit in, I just didn't. I was weird—at least, others told me I was and I believed them. I was weird because I wore matching dresses and jackets made by my mother's deft needle while others wore jeans made by Gloria Vanderbilt, I was weird because I took *Rabrindra Sangeet* singing lessons on the weekends instead of ballet, I was weird because my skin was darker than the color of a melted Hershey bar, I was weird because my name was. I figured, the fewer friends I had, the less I would have to hear my name spoken out loud.

"Alison." I keep my voice as even as I can, even though my palms are sweating. I sit on my clenched fists, in which I hold my true emotions. "No one thinks you're weird. A lot of kids we talk to have unusual experiences. We're just here to find out what's going on with you." From in between my clenched fingers escapes the fact that I do think the little girl is more than a little weird. I stuff the escaped thought back into my fist.

"My parents are mad at me because of the pictures I draw," she says, suddenly matter-of-fact, shrugging her shoulders in a gesture resembling that of any misunderstood preteen. But I have spoken to Alison's parents, and I know that there is more than mere preadolescent angst at work here.

At further prompting, Alison continues, "I'm a fairly sophisticated artist." I notice my attending repressing a smile even as I do the same. Despite all of her concerns about our laughing at her, Alison does not seem to notice. "I've been drawing pictures of creatures, magical creatures, for a while now. But my parents don't like them. They rip up my drawings and send me to my room without dinner. They don't understand me."

As recent immigrants from India, my parents tried to instill in me a strong sense of heritage and culture. They based much of their socialization in the Indian community, taking me to *pujas*, dance recitals, festivals, and functions. They regaled me with stories about "home," and took me on frequent visits to Calcutta. Unfortunately, they could not understand what it meant for me to be both American and Indian. Like other second-generation Indian Americans, I often found myself belonging neither here nor there and having no role models to emulate. During my slightly rebellious high-school years, my mother would condemn me with the epithet, "You're becoming more and more American every day." That statement was particularly painful, since being "American" meant being everything my family was not. It meant allying with the "outsiders" who, more often than not, were alienating, if not outright racist, to my family. Yet, I was obviously not wholly Indian either. Although, during my more difficult days in the U.S., I dreamed of India as a benevolent homeland awaiting me with open arms, during my many vacations in Calcutta I was often considered no more than a "foreigner." It made for a schizophrenic cultural identity, trapped between my parents' nostalgic homeland and my own reluctant one.

"Where do you get the ideas to draw these magical creatures?" I ask, feeling myself on the right track. "Are these images you saw in a book or something?"

Alison scratches her unruly mane of coarse brown curls. "Oh, no," she says, suddenly animated. "I draw the demons I see all around me. I draw the demons that follow me around." She glances over my shoulder, and I resist the impulse to turn around. I can almost feel fire-breath on the back of my neck.

Alison continues, her speed picking up as she rolls her words together. "Theones withtheeightsidedwings, those are the ones that Idraw. I neverdraw cupids or cutsiestuff-likethat, no I never draw stuff like that you know on Valentine's Day I was so sick of those cutsie little cupids with their whiteskin and pinksmiles 'cause life just isn't like that, you know? It's so fake and justallaboutHallmark making up these ideas *they want us to believe in, to make us forget that we're really damned and that there aren't cupids, but* demons *allaroundus, and I'm so sick of those lies and I thought I would just draw the demons, theoneswith- eightsidedwings, like this-this-this," she gesticulates in the air with her finger, outlining what looks to me, in my air- imagination, like the wings of cartoon gargoyles. "I'm very good at capturing what they look like, I'm very inter- ested in how their wings are structured with bones and tendons and how they can fly and all."*

Like every medical student taking psychiatry, I began to name my childhood experiences during my child and adolescent psychiatry rotation. One name I learned was anxiety. I realized that I had many classic examples from my own childhood: the numerous nights I would crouch, nightgown-clad and shivering, on the upstairs landing of our house just so that I could hear my parents' voices and reassure myself they had not abandoned me; the funny rituals I would make up that went way beyond "step on a crack, break your mother's back" (I had to hold my breath, touch the floor three times with my eyes closed and then blow to the leftmost corner of the ceiling every time I left the house or something bad might happen to my family); the insomnia I would suffer all night before any new or unfamiliar event—soaked in sweat, my heart and mind racing, my thoughts panicky. Looking back, I realize that my external demons had burrowed themselves deep into my childhood internal psyche.

* * *

"Do they ever speak to you, the demons?" I ask. "Or do they speak about you to each other?" It's one of the classic questions I have been taught to ask psychiatric patients. True schizophrenics are often the objects of their hallucinations' discussions.

"Oh they talk about me all the time, they're very mean and gossipy." Alison's expression is serious, and I realize that her parents were not exaggerating when they said how bright and precocious Alison used to be before her gradual decline. Her speckled brown eyes are brimming now with water. "They talk about my ugly skin. They talk about my ugly brown skin and how dirty and ugly they think I am." As she speaks, the little girl rubs at her light brown skin, which is two shades lighter than my own, but familiar to me just the same, because Alison shares the delicious nutty color of my mother's complexion. I feel a bitter taste in my mouth and have to fight back my own tears. How she hates what she is, what I am. How she hates what I have finally learned to love.

When I was young, I did not have any nonwhite beauty images. If my expectations of female beauty were Barbie- and Brady Bunch–based, my expectations of male attractiveness were all white and muscle-bound. During the teenage and college years, when I rediscovered the strength of my heritage, I vowed never to look beyond my own community for a life partner. It would be a betrayal of Indian men, of men of color, for me to marry a white man. It would be, I thought at the time, a betrayal of my very heritage. I did not think I could raise Indian children with a non-Indian spouse. And so, when I first met my future husband, I could not imagine that our Anatomy class–inspired romance would lead to marriage. Although his parents were immigrants like mine, they were white professional immigrants from Europe. Of course, I thought at the time, I could not allow myself to marry such a man.

"I wish I could just wash myself off. I really feel like my life would be so much easier if I weren't biracial. I just hate the fact that my mother's black." Alison's final comment is like a punch in my stomach: "I just think that white people and black people shouldn't get married, they shouldn't have kids. It makes it so hard for the kids. It makes the kids so ugly."

Through numerous battles both internal and external, I have come to accept and celebrate the intercultural family I am forming. My children will be brown and yet not brown, Indian and yet not Indian. They will have their own demons, their own battles, their own struggles both social and personal. I know they will have to fight their demons in their own way. All I hope is that I give them the skills to do so and emerge victorious.

"We're going to give you some medicine to help you, Alison," my attending physician says. After the little girl is gone, the psychiatrist's eyes grow worried. "I hope she is not heading toward schizophrenia. That's a road from which there's not much turning back."

My experiences with Alison made me furious, and frustrated, and deeply discouraged. There are, I realized, some demons that are worse than others, some demons that are still unconquerable. Since I have fought my own childhood demons through introspection, debate, and writing, it is terrifying to think that some demons, such as Alison's, attack an individual's very intellect. Her tiny face, terrorized by demons both psychiatric and social, continues to haunt me.

Love in the Afternoon

Flabby bottoms, dangling earlobes, loose skin that bobs and sways beneath the arm: hardly the stuff of sexual fantasies. At least, that's what the media and social norms tell us. The smell of Preparation H is not supposed to inspire passion. If it's not a hard, summer-tanned body, it's just not sexy. Right? Well, it took an afternoon on the Sexual Behaviors Consultation Unit during my psychiatry clerkship to convince me otherwise.

As part of the psychiatry clerkship at Hopkins, students get to spend one afternoon with psychologists and therapists who deal with relationship problems, paraphilias, and other noncriminal complications of normal human sexuality. The afternoon I was assigned to the unit, I was paired off with a female psychiatry resident (who was, just to set the stage, dressed in an enormous flowered dress and about eight months' pregnant at the time), while the male medical student, a rather thin, simpering, bespectacled fellow, was paired off with an equally thin, simpering, and bespectacled male psychiatry resident. Thus gender segregated, we split off to interview the male and female members of an engaged couple.

"They're each sixty-seven," our attending psychiatrist had briefed us, her close-cropped silvery hair and elegant business suit making her the least Dr. Ruth-y sex therapist I had ever seen, "and they're having some sort of sexual problem." She had continued, her silvery voice matching her shining locks, "I expect it's a problem with erectile function, which is quite common in elderly men. Your job is to find out if he's having a problem with just that, or if it's with ejaculation, too."

The four of us kept perfectly straight faces, the pencil-thin men diligently scribbling notes, the flowered, pregnant woman placidly eating a chocolate eclair, and I mesmerized by my attending's glittering diamond earrings while I desperately tried to hide my inner shock. My problem was twofold. The first was just with the idea that a grandparent had sex at all. When I was a little girl learning about the birds and the bees, I had, after hearing about the complicated mechanics, asked my mother seriously, "So you go to a doctor's office to do this?" Although that misconception was eventually cleared up, I guess I continued to allow it to apply for older people. Grandparents didn't have sex like other people, I assumed. They had, at some point in their life, gone, if not into a doctor's office, at least, into some otherworldly state, and engaged in the necessary act of procreation. They didn't enjoy it, of course. And they certainly didn't do it once they reached that asexual, golden stage of retirement. The most fun they had as senior citizens was going to the movies for half price, playing mah-jongg, or enjoying a really scrumptious early-bird special.

My second problem was with the sexual behavior consultation unit in general. From the stories I had heard from my classmates, I had expected to be interviewing someone resembling a guest of Sally Jesse Raphaël: a cross-dressing business executive, a transsexual prostitute, or at least a shoe salesman obsessed with ladies' pumps. I was quite looking forward to the sensationalistic experience. (To be truthful, I was thinking that it would be fodder for a great story.) But instead of some lascivious tale with which to regale my closest friends and relatives, I was to interview Grandma and Grandpa Can't-Keep-It-Up. Big deal, I thought to myself, the most exciting thing that would happen from such a case is a prescription for local testosterone injections, or maybe a penile pump. They were probably some red-faced, rickety old pair who would be horrified to see such young doctors, and use apologetic euphemisms like "male organ," "in an intimate way," and "married activities." I was to be proved very wrong.

Before she sent us on our way, the attending tapped a manicured nail on her clipboard and said, "Remember, if these folks are widowed, they are probably suffering from a lot of grief and clinging to each other as companions in old age. It's quite common, in fact, for elderly men who have lost their wives to feel so guilty about taking a new partner that they can't achieve erections with them."

And with that piece of advice, we were off. The skinny doppelgänger twins in one direction, me and my chocolate-lipped pregnant resident in another. I took a big breath before opening the interview room door. I didn't want to startle the aproned, white-haired, gingerbread-baking, arthritic biddy who was surely to be our interviewee.

I needn't have worried. The woman behind the door, although white haired, and perhaps a sometime baker of gingerbread, was hardly what anyone would call an old biddy. She was instead an elegant, comfortable, and not embarrassed in the least sixty-seven-year-old woman, who looked about ten years younger than she was.

"How are you today?" she asked with ease. "Please, please, have a seat."

The resident and I smiled faintly at each other and did as we were bid. "Why don't you tell us about what brings you here?" the resident began. I sat back quietly. As I knew, I was to be only an observer in this interview, not an active participant.

The patient, whose name was Sylvia, had only just begun her tale when we were interrupted by a shrill beep. The resident apologized to our patient and picked up the phone. "Oh, God!" she exclaimed at whatever news the receiver was telling her, and then, having hung up the phone, explained, "A patient of mine is being admitted to the hospital for attempted suicide. She won't talk to anyone but me. I'm sorry ma'am, but I'm going to have to run to the emergency room for a minute. But," and here, she gestured to me with a confident smile, making my stomach drop about a foot, "this doctor will be happy to finish taking your history. We're a team, so she'll fill me in later." With a pleading look at me, the eclair-eater was sailing out of the room, her flowered dress billowing behind her.

And so it was just Sylvia and me. She looked at me, her sea-blue eyes calm and trusting, matching quite perfectly the sailor suit–inspired sweater and shorts outfit she was sporting. Sylvia patted her no-nonsense short coif with her square-cut, nonmanicured hands and smiled reassuringly.

"Um, why don't you go on?" I suggested. "You were telling me about the first time you had sex." I gulped inwardly, trying to swallow the ominous feeling that the long hand of my own Granny would appear, at any

minute, around the globe from India to slap her impu-
dent granddaughter. Rather than Sylvia, it was me who
was red-faced at the cultural impropriety of asking a
grandmother to tell me about her sex life. If I wasn't
reincarnated as a cockroach for this sin, I thought, I
would surely be damned for taking notes.

But Sylvia didn't seem to mind, and told me her story
with the same no-nonsense style with which she dressed.
She had been brought up in a conservative New England
town, she explained to me, and although she had
engaged in petting and necking (at these words, I was
quite grateful my dark skin was hiding my blush) with
other young men, the first man she had sex with was her
husband. "Well," she admitted with a rueful grin, "my
husband-to-be, at that time."

From her first premarital sexual encounter ("quite
fine," she said, "but it really did get better over time"),
through thirty-nine years of marriage ("at the end there,
my husband was rather ill, so we didn't have intercourse," Sylvia explained sweetly, "but of course I did
continue to perform fellatio"), through her husband's
death, Sylvia told me her whole tale. "And so I've never
had sex with anyone except my husband. Until Walter,
that is," she concluded matter-of-factly.

I felt as winded as if I had run a marathon. But I perse-
vered on, sending desperate telepathic signals for my
resident to return soon. "And how would you describe
the problem you're having with Walter now?" I asked.

"Oh, it's not really me, it's him," she started.

So, my attending had been right, I concluded to myself, the old guy can't get it up. "Oh, so he's having a
problem with his erections?" I suggested helpfully.

Sylvia looked uncomprehendingly at me for a moment. "Oh, no!" she exclaimed in a peal of giggles. "Walt can keep it up for hours!"

I was mystified, and more than a little horrified. "Really?" I asked. How much testosterone did the old guy have?

"Oh, yes," Sylvia reassured me proudly. "You see, Walt uses those penile injections and they work wonders. He's very, very stiff for a very long time."

I felt like I was in the Twilight Zone. But Sylvia, my charming, elegant, grandmotherly patient, was not using those adjectives to discuss lemon meringue, but her partner's "male organ." I took a big breath and struggled on.

"So what exactly is the problem, ma'am?" I asked.

"Oh, we have a wonderful sex life, you see," she told me warmly. "He really gives me quite a lot of pleasure."

I really didn't want to ask it, but had been trained to do so. "You can achieve orgasm?" I tried to ask without flinching.

"Multiple ones. They just go on and on," Sylvia told me, her face beaming gently. She was as proud as if she were describing a grandchild's spelling-bee performance. "Better than I've ever had in my whole life. Much better than with my husband. I feel like I'm always sexually aroused with Walt. He's a wonderful lover."

My shock was overcome by how impressed I was. I was dying to meet this Walt. "But you haven't told me what the problem is, Sylvia," I reminded her.

Sylvia nodded, back on track. "Oh, I feel terrible because it's always me coming. I orgasm so much, and all the time, but Walt, well, to put it bluntly, well, he never comes at all. I keep trying and trying to make him come, but he just outlasts me every time. Even if we have sex all day, he won't come. I just don't know what to do about it."

And there it was. Not a problem with erections, since Walt and Sylvia had already discovered the miracles of localized testosterone injections, but ejaculation. The resident finally came back to finish up the interview, filling in Sylvia's unremarkable medical, psychiatric, social, and occupational history. And with all the paperwork done, we were ready to interview the couple together. We were ready to meet the indefatigable Walt.

I don't know what I was expecting. Perhaps not the rickety mah-jongg-playing old-timer of my earlier stereotypes, but at least a reserved elderly gentleman as cultured as Sylvia. It certainly wasn't what I got.

"Hey, there, Docs!" Walt boomed when—having reconvened with the emaciated male team and our elegantly attired attending—we five white-coated clinicians traipsed into the room where Sylvia and Walt were now waiting together. He was a ruddy-faced, big-boned man, whose beefy nose looked as if it had seen one or two fights. His broad knuckles engulfed Sylvia's elegantly tapered hands in what looked like a callousy embrace. His khaki shorts and shirt, which were probably bought at the shopping mall by Sylvia, didn't make him look anything like a big-game hunter back from Kenyan safari. Instead, he looked like a brawny man from the docks unused to owning clothes that weren't denim. His watery eyes were a little dissipated, but bright and lively. And they were brimming with an intense love for the genteel woman perched beside him.

"The first thing I gotta tell you docs, just like I told the fellas before"—Walt nodded at the skinny male team, who looked like the least likely candidates to be called "fella" by even an elderly man exuding so much masculinity—"is that I am crazy—crazy—about this here woman. This here lady," he amended. Walt's face turned almost purple with emotion, while the placid Sylvia's face only tinted a slight pink. "I love her to death," he added, as if we hadn't gotten the message before.

"Oh, Walt, now, hush," the object of his affection scolded lightly.

"No, Sylvie, I just want 'em to know how much I love ya. I want 'em to know that our problem doesn't have anything to do with how I feel about ya. To me," Walt told us, "this is the most beautiful, sexy woman in the world." He turned passionately to her, "Hell, I would come all day with ya if I could, Sylvie. You know that, darlin'. I would come all day for you."

The pregnant resident, who had been filled in only briefly on what she had missed, looked shocked. The male med student and resident, now more mirror images of each other than ever, were hunched over notebooks, taking notes. "Male patient declares much emotion for female patient," I imagined them writing, "and would ejaculate all day for her if he could."

"So, why don't you tell us about your history, Walt," the attending asked, "since this issue seems primarily to originate with you. That way, we can fully understand the context behind it."

"What d'ya wanna know, Doc?"

"Why don't you tell me about how you grew up, Walter?" she prompted, picking a piece of imaginary lint off her lapel. "Tell us about your first sexual experiences."

"Well, I grew up pretty poor. My daddy worked at a mine in Pennsylvania, and we lived, our whole family, in one room. We shared a bathroom and kitchen with three other families from the mine," Walt explained. Even the scribbling men stopped their writing to look up. It was a pretty different upbringing from most of us.

"Go on," the attending urged.

"Since it was such close quarters, ya know, ya saw a lot of stuff pretty young," Walt said dryly. "I saw the next-door-neighbor girls naked in the bathroom all the time." Sylvia looked undisturbed, listening to what was obviously a story she had heard before. "By the time I was twelve, I was havin' sex with 'em in the bathroom."

"Really?" our attending's voice was smooth as silk. "Tell us about that."

Walt's gravelly voice was in stark contrast. "What's there to tell?" he guffawed pleasantly. "It was pretty amazing to be gettin' so much action so young."

Someone snickered. It might have been me.

Our attending continued, unfazed. "Hmm . . ." she said thoughtfully, "tell us about your contraceptive choices."

This time it was Walt's turn to snicker. "Choices?" he boomed. "I didn't know about any choices—except rubbers. My dad found out I was so active and gave me a condom drawer at home. But then I would run through them so quick that he opened up an account for me at the corner pharmacy."

Walt told us about his remarkable youth first working in the mines, then on the docks of Baltimore. He described his multiple sexual liaisons, his extensive experiences with prostitutes, and his extracurricular activity outside of his thirty-year marriage.

"My wife, she had some infection or somethin' down there for a while," Walter explained vaguely, "and after that, I just couldn't bring myself to have sex with her. I would go down on her and all, but I just didn't like to have sex with her anymore. And then she got cancer, just like Sylvie's husband did, and that was that."

"And you feel guilty about that?" the attending suggested helpfully, ready to prove her theory about widowers, guilt, and sexual dysfunction.

"Nah, not really," Walter replied, swiping his nose absentmindedly with the back of a broad hand. "I feel bad that she died, but it wasn't really my fault or nothin'. And it was a long time ago. Besides which, it's not like I didn't tell her I was foolin' around on her. I did. I would never fool around on someone and not tell them." Here, he turned and grasped Sylvia's hand in both his enormous paws. "But I would never fool around on this lady. No, ma'am, never. There ain't no need. We can talk about anything, everything. I can tell her whatever's on my mind. It was never this way with my wife. I guess Sylvie's just always been the one for me."

Sylvia, who had been demurely listening, suddenly piped up. "This is the best, most open relationship that either of us has ever been in," she said earnestly. "It's as if our marriages were just practice runs for the real thing."

Walt patted her hand, his eyes hazy. "I guess it's better late than never."

The attending psychologist looked a little perplexed. "So what is the problem you are having?"

"We have a great sex life, Doc, we really do," Walter assured her, with Sylvia nodding in agreement beside him. "Two, three times a day usually, we're at it. She wakes me up in the middle of the night, wantin' it, and I love it!" His ruddy face glowed with rapture. "I could give this woman oral sex until kingdom come." Sylvia grinned coyly at her adoring partner.

My pregnant resident looked, large-eyed, at me. I tried not to grin at Walter's unintentional pun. The attending pushed onward. "But what about intercourse?"

"Well, ma'am, that's the thing," Walter admitted ruefully. "Like I told the fellas here, I can keep my little guy up for a long, long time. Yep, he's a real trooper." The fellas looked blankly confused. "But he just won't do his thing. I just can't have an orgasm with Sylvie, even though I really want to."

"Can you achieve orgasm when she's giving you oral sex, or when she's manually masturbating you?" In her crisp, professional tones, our attending made the most intimate sexual experiences sound strangely dry-cleaned.

"Nope. Not at all," Walter baldly admitted. "It's not that it's not nice—it is—but the water never rushes the dam."

Walter's colorful metaphors were clearly something Sylvia was used to. She added helpfully, "He tells me he can have an orgasm when he's by himself. And also, well . . ." Here she paused and looked at her now silent partner.

"Yes?" the pregnant resident prompted, speaking for all of us. We were hooked, and wanted to hear the rest of their intimate story.

With a quick look at Walter, Sylvia finished the sentence. "When I turn my back to him."

"Excuse me?" The clinical team was a little flabbergasted.

Walter jumped in, explaining, "My little guy does a great job when I'm alone. You know how it is, fellas," he said in a warm tone of male bonding. The gesture fell a little short. While the male resident tried to nod reassuringly at the patient, the medical student just looked thunderstruck, as if his innermost secrets had been found out. Walter continued, jovially, "I got a particular grip I like, a stroke, a timing. It's all pretty one-two-three." Here, Walter added some rather colorful hand gestures, which did nothing to calm my medical student colleague's discomfiture. He coughed twice, gulped, and coughed again.

The attending came to his rescue with a change of subject. "Have you ever tried to show her," she asked, "your grip, your timing, your—" the attending ran her finger lightly over a bemused mouth, "one-two-three?"

"I can't," Walter admitted ruefully. "It just seems like a waste of time. Why should I bother this pretty lady with that kind of stuff? I'm happy just making her happy."

Sylvia's voice broke in quietly. "I've always wanted you to show me, Walt. I just didn't know how to ask."

Her fiancé squirmed even more than the male medical student. "Aw, honey," he mumbled to the floor, "don't ask me that."

The attending tried another angle. "Were you able to achieve orgasm with anyone else recently?" she asked, perhaps tactfully trying to discover the extent of Walter's extracurricular jauntings.

"No. It's not like I didn't get it on with a lot of ladies after my wife died," Walter explained slowly, "I did. But I just couldn't come with them, either. I guess the difference is, none of them ever seemed to care about it." He cheered considerably then, his eyes bright as he gazed at his lover. "My Sylvie, she won't stand for my little soldier not doin' his duty," he finished proudly.

"Hmm." The psychologist tapped her peach-colored nails delicately on her clipboard. "And what's this about Sylvia turning her back to you?"

The overtly unabashable Walter was again tongue-tied. "Well, that's kinda silly, see . . ." he started slowly.

His partner didn't let him finish, and he gazed up from the floor gratefully at the interruption. Sylvia was as calm as if she were describing a simple pie recipe to an eighth grader. "Walt is a little embarrassed, but he shouldn't be. You see, he can only orgasm in my presence if I have my back turned to him. I'll turn away and he'll masturbate off the side of the bed."

There was a stunned silence. The male medical student looked as if he was going to jump out of his skin. The woman resident flared her nostrils expressively in my direction.

"Do you think, Walter, that turning your back isn't as bad as teaching Sylvia how you would like her to arouse your, er," the attending coughed delicately, "little soldier?"

Walt sat in silence for a moment. The answer had always lain in his heart, but talking it over seemed to strengthen his resolve. Finally, pulling Sylvia's slight frame into a bearlike embrace, he said, "Sure." His voice was teary and muffled from within her hair. She patted him tenderly on the back. "Anything for Sylvie," he added simply.

And that was that. With some negotiation about future counseling, and some hearty reassurance, our chic attending was done with her treatment.

As we were gathering our things to leave, Walter had some parting advice for the fellas. "It only gets better from here, guys," he said, his macho guffaw back in place, "as long as you remember that playin' with yourself is never as fun as playin' soldiers with a lady friend."

The male resident gave him an entirely goofy thumbs-up sign while the medical student scurried out of the room, pushing me aside to do so.

The elegant attending, the waddling resident, and I exchanged grins. Old age had been given quite a different spin for us that afternoon. We had a lot to look forward to.

Not Just Skin Deep

I'm terribly ugly.

It's an awful statement, a sentence that has meaning beyond superficial appearance. It's a statement filled with self-loathing and self-hate. Unfortunately, it's a statement that I have made to reflected images of myself. It's also a statement that I've heard other women make, women who were all ostensibly attractive, if not stunning.

Yes, beauty standards are changing. Madison Avenue, long considered the source of American, and for that matter international, women's angst is catching up with reality. Instead of only the waif Kate Moss, the large-size model Emme is now plastered all over Times Square. Instead of only Barbie, there are dark-skinned dollies crowding the shelves at F.A.O. Schwarz. Instead of the unrealistically bouncy Charlie's Angels, we have the ever-so-realistic female role models of—*Baywatch*? Well, at least we have the ditzy post-feminist Ally McBeal.

Why do I bring this up? What in the world can this have to do with medicine? A lot of women have low self-esteem, right? Well, yes. But as I've gone through my medical training, I've come to learn that certain kinds of low self-esteem are more dangerous than others, certain self-loathing more pathological.

Take, for instance, a story that is plastered all over news headlines these days: neonaticide. The cases are oddly similar—teenage girls who hide their unplanned and unwanted pregnancies and eventually have some part in, if not the death, at least the disposal of their secretly delivered newborn babies. From Delaware to Florida to Texas, these accused baby killers are almost exactly the same—model daughters devastated at the thought of disappointing their loving parents; perfectionists who must erase any memory of their fall from grace; little girls horrified at the responsibility that comes with their newly adult bodies. This too is self-loathing—a loathing of the woman a girl is becoming, a loathing of her own sexuality, a loathing of the prospect of imperfection. It is a loathing so strong that it is able to disguise a pregnant body, preventing it from gaining weight. It is a loathing so strong that it is able to black out an enormous reality. It is a loathing so strong that it destroys another life without fully understanding the implications.

As a medical student, I have often argued that the key to averting devastating situations like these is prevention: access to family planning, health education, and abortion. We must give young women all the opportunities they need to make healthy choices. And yet, opportunity does not automatically confer the self-confidence needed to make appropriate decisions. Contraception alone cannot help a young woman make the transition into adulthood with safety.

The cases of neonaticide recently in the news remind me, inexorably, of gymnasts, ice skaters, child models—the prepubescent creatures American society holds up as icons of womanhood. They remind me, ultimately, of the skeletal little anorexic girls I saw during my psychiatry rotation. These are the ones who swallowed—lock, stock, and barrel—the message that beauty can only be achieved by arresting aging; that adult womanhood is incompatible with attractiveness. Instead of killing their babies, they slowly killed themselves.

I once took care of an eleven-year-old anorexic. So much younger than the adolescent girls, she was moved from the regular anorexia and bulimia unit to the children's psychiatry ward. It seemed that by hanging out with the older anorexics, she was only learning their bad habits, getting advice about how to more expertly hide her food from the eagle-eye nurses, how to exercise in the shower, how to use laxatives to rid her body of pounds. And so, I came to take care of her while on my child and adolescent psychiatry rotation. She was the most pathetic sight I have ever seen. An enormous head balanced awkwardly on a pinlike body, skin grotesquely dry and taut over sinew and bone, eyes huge in an infantile face. To add to the spectacle, she would parade around the floor in over-tight tank tops and cut-off shorts, wiggling her bony behind and batting her eyelashes in what I can only assume was her eleven-year-old idea of outrageous flirtation with every male staff member. One day, after learning that many anorexics have self-concepts years younger than their actual age, I asked my young patient a rather telling question.

"If you could be any age, any age at all," I had asked, "how old would you be?"

Without batting an eyelash, the eleven-year-old gave me a horrifying answer. "Oh, that's easy," she said. "I would be five. I have never been as happy as I was back then."

It was almost as absurd as if she had told me she wanted to be back in the womb. And yet, this same girl who yearned for infancy was manifesting a disease far older than her years. Indeed, for the rest of her hospitalization, she continued to badger our team about allowing her to move to the adult anorexia unit.

Her parents were of no help. "She's far more mature than her years," her mother had argued.

"I wanna hang out with the big girls," the daughter had whined.

And yet, she wanted to be five. It was a logical mobius loop.

I realized then that I have never in my life wanted to be younger than I am. When I was eleven, I dreamed of being sweet sixteen—an age, I assumed, that would bring true love, success, and marriage. While my notions weren't exactly accurate, they did reflect something that my little patient was lacking: a hope that something better in life was yet to come.

The odd thing is, this lack of hope for the future was so profound in my young patient that she did not have an age-appropriate way to express it. She had to reach into that dreaded future to find a disease grown-up enough to convey her fear of growing up.

It wasn't that I didn't have my own self-esteem problems as a child. I quite freely admit that I, too, suffered from a shockingly low self-concept. And as a child of color, a daughter of immigrants, I had the additional burden of dark skin, a foreign name, and "bizarre" customs that were the favorite target of schoolyard ridicule. "Hindoo go home," I heard more than once. I can only assume they meant some fanciful home in South Asia, since my real birthplace was no more exotic than Columbus, Ohio. Indeed, race is yet another complicating factor that is thrown on social expectations about women's sexualities and bodies. My own experience is that, as with most women of color, the worst racist insults I've faced were aimed at my looks, my body, and as I grew older, my sexuality.

For women of color, beauty is indeed far more complex than a reflected image. Our beauty has long been used as a racist weapon against us. So the African American woman's hair is too kinky, her nose too flat, her skin too dark; she is either the asexual "mammy" or the hypersexual primitive beast. The Latina is too dark, too "loose," too lazy, too stupid, while the East Asian woman is either the demure, self-sacrificing Madame Butterfly or the seductive sex kitten eager to please. Similarly, the images used against women of my community, South Asians, are just as vicious: The South Asian woman is either the foreign, smelly, pagan, primitive, sari-swathed creature, or she is the sultry, long-haired, nose-ringed sex goddess. I myself have directly faced these images; as a teenager in white America, I was a wallflower who only wanted to be swallowed up by the ground at parties. By the time I reached college, I was a campus exotic—desired for my foreign looks, my mysterious ways. Only recently, when I and a South Asian woman friend walked into a New York restaurant, an entire row of martini-guzzling investment bankers at the bar turned to seductively singsong at us, "KA-MA SU-TRA!" Barring the unlikely possibility they were Indophilic scholars who shouted out the names of ancient love texts whenever they had too much vodka in them, these men were clearly exemplifying the fascination that mainstream America has with "exotic" images, and the ease at which these stereotypic notions are put upon real women.

These external forces must, of course, be understood in context. The cohort of South Asians to which I belong, children of the primarily white-collar post-1965 immigrants from India, has, in not so many words, made sexuality their issue. This group of immigrants has now been in the United States for more than thirty years, and so their American-born children are now in young adulthood. Yet sexuality is not discussed openly. It is ostensibly taboo, and "hard topics" such as AIDS, contraception, and homosexuality are hardly brought up unless in tones of condemnation. For South Asian communities, "dating," "prom," and "arranged marriages" are the rubric under which sexuality is brought to the forefront and hotly debated—over dining room tables, long distance phone calls, and "youth" or "second generation" forums at community conferences. Sexuality is ultimately at the forefront of intergenerational interaction, and young women, who are often considered the preservers of all that is "traditional" in food, clothing, dress, and custom, may in fact, be faced with the option of not carrying out their sexual choices or being labeled cultural betrayers by their parents and communities. They are torn between two cultures, and as the communities present it, being South Asian means being respectful, loving daughters, while being American stands for everything from disrespect to debauchery. Thus, South Asian women form their sexual self-concepts in an environment that is, at times, both internally and externally hostile. There are no role models, no forums in which to frankly air fears. And so, confusion, repression, racism, and the generic low self-esteem of youth gets turned inward, often to devastating consequences.

There was another young woman I met while on psychiatry, this time during my adult rotation. Every Friday during this clerkship, there was a conference with the chairman of the department where an interesting patient was presented to a roomful of residents. One week, the conference was quite a shock for me. For the first time in my medical school career, the patient who shuffled shyly into the room full of white-coated strangers was a second-generation South Asian woman—like me. The history, which I have abbreviated and am altering for obvious reasons of confidentiality, went something like this (try to imagine it being read in the driest of monotones in front of the patient while she passively, helplessly, listens to herself being described):

Lila Prasad is a twenty-four-year-old woman who was being seen in the outpatient psychiatry clinic after having been in the hospital three months previously. She was born and raised in the United States Midwest, the youngest daughter of Indian immigrants. There was no abuse in her childhood and she describes her relationship with her parents as healthy and supportive. She has two older sisters, one a lawyer and one with an MBA. By the time Lila went to a respected, private East Coast college, it was expected she would be the family doctor. Yet, her grades weren't up to snuff, and upon graduation, Lila was planning on working for a few years and then applying to grad school.

It was at her college graduation that her mother noticed there was something wrong. Lila, who is 5' 4", had shrunk from her regular 110 pounds to 90 pounds. "It's just finals, Mom," she had explained. Yet, in the ensuing months, there was no excuse as Lila's weight went down to 85, 80, 75, and finally 70 pounds. In short, Lila was hospitalized with anorexia nervosa, starving herself almost to the point of death.

The interesting thing about Lila's interview, for me, was my reactions to her versus the roomful of other, primarily white, resident physicians' reactions. As soon as she walked in, I wanted to pick her up and run away. She was a gaunt, grim-expressioned, dead-eyed thing—yet she looked like every one of the South Asian women I have ever known. I could almost imagine her in a glittery silk *salwaar kamese*, bedecked and bejeweled, chattering away at an Indian community function. But she wasn't. She was in a roomful of physicians asking her an endless series of questions. As they continued their interviews, it became clear that Lila's anorexia did not stem from the morbid "fear of fatness" that is the hallmark of most anorexics, but the deep-seated, horribly strong belief that she was ugly.

"Don't you want to get married?" the psychiatry chairman asked her. While I thought his question a bit heterosexist—Lila very well might have been attracted to women—I also thought that he had hit the nail, if albeit awkwardly, on the head.

In South Asian communities, marriage is a central landmark of family life; it is the key transition into adulthood. In these cultures, marriage and sexuality are traditionally separated, with the former being associated with families and communities and responsibility, and the latter being considered a private, personal experience. However, with immigration and Westernization, romantic notions of marriage have altered the traditional construct. Of course, whether you pick out your own spouse or have one arranged, South Asian families usually still expect children to get married.

Lila's answer to the attending's question was telling. "No," she replied abruptly, staring at an undeterminable spot on the carpet. "I'm just out of the running." Her face was still and calm even as she said, "Don't you see that I'm ugly? I've always been ugly."

I did not. And yet, I did see how she loathed herself. And as the roomful of psychiatrists asked her if she felt her anorexia was a way she could control her body, I wondered if it wasn't just a way that she had found, as I had wished so many times in childhood, to make her brown-skinned body disappear.

When she left, the chairman laughed in a paternal, understanding way. "How could she think that she was ugly? Why, she's as cute as a button!"

How could I explain it all? It was just too complicated, and I'm not sure there is a DSM-IV category for cultural traditions, community pressures, or internalized racism.

Medicine categorizes illness, but it does not always understand it. Lila's condition could hardly be investigated with X-ray, microscope, or even thorough psychiatric interview. Indeed, she was not that different from the baby anorexic I cared for, from the girls on the news for killing their own babies. All of these young women are impacted by forces larger than medical ones. Whether purging themselves of calories, babies, or just overwhelming cultural standards, these girls are turning their disappointment at their own imperfection into hatred of themselves.

Race, gender, and sexuality are issues that are oftentimes ignored in medicine, despite the fact that they strongly inform many medical conditions. For me, writing, speaking, and taking action about these issues must go hand-in-hand with my career as a physician. Through our collective introspection, analysis, and activism, we bring forth a beauty that too many young women do not see in the mirror. We bring forth a beauty that is more than skin deep, a beauty that emerges from recognizing the forces at work around us and learning to name them.

Lady Doctor

One of the things I like the most about India is the way it jostles your sense of perspective. Not subtly, but in the harshest, most shocking way, the ancient country of my foreparents brings together contradictions, questions one's understanding of reality, and challenges each and every visitor to her shores to more deeply understand their place in the universe. I see no better metaphor for the emotional journey that is a trip to India than a harrowing jaunt down her all-too-crowded urban roads. Narrowly avoiding taxi, rickshaw, cow, goat, human, buffalo, and metallic-horn-screeching bus, the visitor to India jostles uncomfortably down pothole-ridden streets, senses overloaded by smells both delicious and revolting, sights both awe-inspiring and demoralizing, and sounds both melodious and cacophonic. The spectacle of creatively spelled vehicle-art adorning the backs of most manmade forms of transport speaks all too well for the experience: "Don't Kees Marrade Bus" admonishes one anti-tailgating slogan; "My India is Grate" declares another nationalistic one. And my favorite tailgate message, painted in swirling letters under a wide-eyed, tongue-waggling painting of the fearsome goddess Kali: "DENGAAR!"

It was to this land of contradictions that I turned, twice, during my medical career, to gather some sense of greater perspective. Well, that wasn't the ostensible reason that either trip was made. The first, taken the summer after my first year of medical school, was under the auspices of what I thought of as my "granny grant"—that is, money to do some research and simultaneously visit my grandmothers in Calcutta. With one of the infectious disease attendings at Hopkins, I had designed a survey to learn about Calcutta physicians' familiarity with HIV and their use of universal precautions. The second trip, a few years later, was a clinical rotation at India's premier medical research institution, The All-India Institute of Medical Sciences (AIIMS), in New Delhi. Not only did I go to AIIMS to see what an international clinical career would be like, I wanted to introduce my then boyfriend (now husband), Boris, to India for the first time. During the first trip, I thought I was going to learn about clean needles and syringes, double gloving, and physicians' perceived self-risk. During the second, I thought I would see esoteric tropical diseases, infections commonplace in India, but utterly absent in my Western medical education. While I won't say that I didn't learn these things, what I gained far more of from both of these experiences was a sense of humor, a sense of my place in medicine, and a greater understanding of myself.

India is an ancient country, where layer upon layer of modern life has been built upon strong-rooted, complex histories of invasion, ethnic diversity, and constant waves of immigration—from the Middle Eastern Moghuls to the Greek troops of Alexander the Great, to the Chinese, Jewish, Portuguese, French, Spanish, and of course, British. The interesting thing about India is that no layer of history completely obliterates, or subsumes, the ones that came before. Modern India, thus, is like an onion that can be peeled away to reveal simultaneously existing realities from different centuries. Cultural nuances, norms, and etiquette are therefore just as complicated. There are things done and other things said, things implied and other things asserted: It's quite different from America, where people pride themselves on looking others in the eye, saying what they mean, and shooting from the hip. I would soon discover that an American, even an Indian American, trying to stumble her way through a cultural system as complicated as India's is like a bull trying to tiptoe through a china shop.

Having grown up in the States, weaned on the ambrosia of my parents' immigrant nostalgia, I had always thought of India as "home"—that I was merely a brown-skinned girl who had somehow become trapped on foreign soil. And so I dealt with childhood racism by convincing myself that there was a country where I would be embraced as a sister, that there was a place halfway around the globe where I did indeed belong. Childhood trips only confirmed these fanciful notions. While I had no relatives with whom to spend holidays in America, India was full to the brim of cheek-squeezing, emotion-overflowing, loud, boisterous, affectionate, spoiling relations. Even strangers on the street looked like me, and seemed to accept my belonging there without question. And so I tried to reinforce these good feelings by blending in utterly, holding my breath to try and prevent any stray Americanism from escaping my lips, trying to discipline gangly limbs to move with the gentle sway of Indian women, curbing my unruly, curious eyes not to stare people straight in the face, as is still my habit, but to look demurely down to the ground. I knew it was this last habit that would always betray me. No matter how I squeezed the rest of myself into an awkward-fitting role, my rebellious eyes would always give me away. And so I trained myself not to let anyone sneak a peek at them.

As I grew older, however, the mask of my Indian-ness grew to be a greater and greater burden every time I visited my grandparents over summer holidays. As a teenager, I discovered that Western dress meant unwanted molestation by strangers on the street—the untoward hand brushing unmentionables as I squeezed through a crowd, a group of vendors staring lasciviously, young men passing obnoxious comments as they sauntered leeringly by. And so, one more layer was added to my disguise, and I began wearing strictly Indian clothes when traveling in my parents' native land. While it didn't solve all my problems, it definitely toned them down. Other issues were about movement. Young women from "nice families" it seems, just don't wander willy-nilly around Indian cities without proper escort. Or at least, that's what my relatives tried to convince me. And I saw proof. My female cousins either took one public transport route from home to office/school/college and back again, or had cars and drivers that took them exactly to and from where they wanted to go. What I didn't realize until later was that most of them were deviating from parental strictures, but secretly, and usually with disapproved of male escorts. I, as a foreign import, a babe in the woods, an "Amreekan," only had my parents as cultural reference points. I wasn't used to the layers of delicate deceptions, veils both real and metaphorical, which Indian women wear to enable their own unmolested mobility. I was used to going where I wanted when I wanted, driving myself, and never needing to lie or deceive anyone about it. I was only asking for trouble by wanting to travel around by myself, my relatives told me. And from the negative experiences I had the few times I tried, I believed them.

At first, on my "granny grant" trip, I tried my damndest to keep up the entire, complicated disguise. But fitting in professionally is quite different from trying to fit in while vacationing. Properly swathed in *salwaar kamese*, driven in a private car by a neighborhood tough guy my grandparents knew, I set out, with one year of medical school beneath my belt—or *dupatta*, in my case—to interview Calcutta physicians about their knowledge, attitudes, and practices regarding HIV and AIDS. It was a little naive of me to think it would be easy.

"Who sent you?" was one of the first questions suspicious-faced male secretaries would ask me when I arrived at my appointments with various medical school department heads.

"I've come from Johns Hopkins with a research project," I would explain in my best "dutiful daughter" Bengali.

They would look at me dubiously. No wonder. I'm sure I didn't look like an American researcher to them. My air of polite trepidation and conservative style made me more closely resemble a precocious convent-schooler than a foreign physician. I would reassure them, without much avail.

"Shouldn't they have sent somebody really from Johns Hopkins?" some would ask, assuming I was some local emissary of the famed American institution.

Others would assume it was a case of mistaken identity. "But I thought Johns Hopkins was in America?" they would warily probe.

Still others were openly unkind. They would challenge, "Are you sure you're a doctor?"

The worst was when they doubted my identity altogether. "Are you a real American, anyway?" I got more than once.

And finally, they would order me to "Sit there," "Come here," or, even more commonly, after walking off and realizing I was still following them, they would turn over their shoulders to command, heavily accented, "Wait, wait."

On one such occasion, when the order to "wait" did not come in time, I had followed a greasy-haired office staffer into the room of the department chair. Like a Nawab from days of old, he was holding court; sitting not on a throne, but on its Indian modern-day equivalent— an imitation leather office chair adorned with the perfunctory Turkish towel, which is the mark of all truly important subcontinental officials (to prevent them, on hot afternoons, from sticking to their seats). I realized why this medical kingpin had been too busy to receive any of my calls—he had a full-fledged campus crisis on his hands.

"And then Dr. Chakrovorty's daughter was seen climbing out the window, slithering down the drainpipe, sir," one obsequious-faced underling was reporting.

"And then?" The medical Nawab's beady eyes glittered excitedly from their sunken position in his fleshy face.

"And then with that young Dr. Sarkar, sir—"another underling rubbed his hands as if savoring a delicious meal—"she ran off—*Hawa!* Vanished!" They were so engrossed in the story, no one even noticed me.

"And Chakrovorty got her back? How?" Nawab-ji was almost slobbering now.

"Alas, Krishna-Radha didn't think about the guards at the gate when they planned their ren-dez-vous," he said, pronouncing every letter of the word. "So they brought them back to the quarters before her father knew she was gone."

Clearly, there are some things that take precedence over day-to-day medical business.

Once I had finally made my way past the office mice-men and their fat cat administrative bosses, my reception wasn't much better. "Double gloves?" doctors would answer scornfully. "We're lucky if we have enough gloves to wear at all."

I would soon see suites in the hospitals that were dedicated solely for the purpose of re-washing and drying disposable latex gloves multiple times. I would see, with my own eyes, needles and syringes being reused—"If they want a fresh needle, the family has to go to the market and buy one themselves," one doctor had explained to me. "But even then, there's nothing to guarantee that the scavengers who go through the hospital trash bins haven't just washed, packaged, and resold dirty needles as new in the market." I would see, day after day, families having to buy medical instruments for use on their ill relations, wash hospital sheets and gowns, gather and transport lifesaving blood for transfusions.

And the staff was more than a little angry about my questions. "AIDS? Do you think that AIDS should be our priority in a country where babies die of diarrhea every day?" one dedicated physician had scolded.

Others were straight-up misinformed. "AIDS is a gay disease, and there is no gay problem here in India," a self-righteous administrator told me, happily ignoring the reality of a large Indian gay and lesbian population, which is in fact growing more visible and vocal.

The best were answers born of paranoia. As a state run by the Communist Party of India-Marxist (CPI-M), West Bengal is historically xenophobic, particularly when it comes to the big bad capitalist baddie, the United States. "How do we know that AIDS is not a CIA plot?" a doctor had ferociously argued with me. "To take our attention away from real problems—poverty, water, food?" There was something about the frenetic tenor of his speech that made me think he suspected me of being a covert operative responsible for distributing harmful propaganda to the Third World.

I soon realized that being a "good Bengali girl" and asking questions about AIDS was incompatible. It took me a while, but by the end of my trip, I was speaking English, which, sadly enough, was the only way I could get in the door at some hospitals, and looking doctors straight in the eye. They still weren't convinced I was from Hopkins, but at least they had stopped patting me on the head.

By the time I took my second jaunt to India, I was not alone, and that made my life complicated in ways that mere Western-style clothes never could. Dating, which is still not publicly "done" in India, provides no social or cultural space. Romantic partnership is recognized solely through marriage, or at least, engagement. Since Boris and I were neither married nor even engaged at the time we ventured to New Delhi to do clinical rotations, I presented him, over the phone to my curious Calcutta relatives, as a "school friend," a classmate who happened to be doing the same clinical course work abroad. But that was hardly the end of my problems. The physicians at AIIMS, like those in Calcutta, were highly doubtful of my status as a Johns Hopkins medical student. Interestingly enough, however, Boris's white skin and clearly Western ethnic heritage gave him the legitimacy that a little brown girl in Indian clothes didn't have. It was a double-edged sword. Since I was clearly traveling around with this white person, it didn't matter how I singsong lilted my accent or how well I dressed in ethnic clothing—I was obviously not a run-of-the-mill Indian woman. Yet, by being with him, my status as a foreign physician in training was fairly secure. It was an uncomfortable, tenuous situation that provided me with more than my share of stress.

"Where are your papers?" Dr. Singh, the rotund, regally manned chairman of pediatrics had bellowed at me the first day I arrived at AIIMS. Indians are notoriously fond of official stamped, notarized, and signed-in-three-places forms, and unfortunately, I did not have the right ones.

"I never received those," I had protested, once I saw which forms he wanted. That only served to incur his demonic wrath even further. As I was soon to learn, the medical hierarchy in India is far more stringent than the one we have in the States. And a department chairman is never, never wrong. Particularly about such auspicious things as forms.

"Don't talk!" Dr. Singh had bellowed, startling me out of my wits. Then, suddenly, he spotted Boris, who was standing a distance behind me.

"You are who?" Dr. Singh had authoritatively asked. I didn't think it was appropriate to correct his grammar right then.

Once Boris had responded, the chairman's demeanor,

while still unpleasant, changed into something a little less glowering. "We expect students will come with appropriate paperwork from the in-is-ti-tution from which they are coming," he explained over my head to Boris.

With the help of my great white knight, I somehow managed to make it through that conversation. Of course, despite the fact that I was the one who was to rotate through pediatrics, I was never directly spoken to throughout the rest of the conversation.

Dr. Singh was not the only meanie at AIIMS. In clinic, the hierarchy was no different. The pediatricians, who are by far the nicest physicians in U.S. hospitals, were actually really abrasive. I suppose it's because the plethora of gastrointestinal and respiratory infectious diseases ravaging children throughout South Asia makes pediatrics a highly competitive and respected field. With this additional glory comes additional snobbery, not unlike surgeons in the U.S.

One afternoon, we were seeing a seven-year-old boy with an abdominal mass. "What is the differential?" the attending had asked me.

I thought it over quickly. Neuroblastoma? No, the child was too old. "Wilms' tumor?" I asked tentatively, then added, "Hemangioblastoma?"

The pediatrician glowered at me. "List the obvious, the usual, first," he scolded.

But I didn't know. I could only shake my head in wonder.

"Come on, the usual, the everyday, the commonplace!" The physician was getting more and more upset, until, finally, he just answered his own question. "Have you ever heard of tuberculosis?"

His sarcasm was in fact warranted, because although

I had seen a few cases of pulmonary TB in the States, I hardly remembered learning about extrapulmonary manifestations of the disease, let alone abdominal growths. "An abdominal mass in a child, unless otherwise explained," the doctor had lectured, as if to a particularly stupid child, "is always tuberculosis."

It would have taken too much energy to explain my own reality.

And my reality, certainly, was quite different from anything we saw in the Indian hospital. The wildlife itself was something astounding. Cockroaches and other breeds of creepie-crawlies were more than common, at least on the ward, which is where less wealthy patients lay, eight to a small room. More startling than the bugs, however, were the various families of large, aggressive monkeys that lived on the roof of the hospital and were occasionally seen scampering down the open-air corridors. They terrorized the families of patients, who, having perhaps come from far-away villages with an ill family member, camped outside on the hospital lawns. Once, a man with a cloth satchel was walking a few steps ahead of us on the lawn when a monkey practically leaped on him, knocking the satchel out of his hands. There was more than one ape that emerged from the woodwork, scampering to get their fill of the oranges and mangoes that spilled out of the bag. Thievery complete in less than a minute, they bolted to the hospital roof, where they rained orange peels upon their cursing victim's head.

Another stark contrast to my reality was the reactions of patients to their doctors. In east Baltimore, patients are sometimes, if not abusive, at least openly aggressive to their caretakers, demanding better food, different medicines, quicker cures. My experience in India was that patients thought of their physicians as gods, and unfortunately, the physicians did nothing to correct their misheld assumption. Doctors rarely explained the details of diseases, procedures, or treatments to patients who were often too awestruck and shy to challenge the "Doctor-Sahib"—or in the women's cases, the "Lady Doctor." Even I, as one of the white-coated professionals, was afforded a respect and honor that almost bordered on the servile.

I remember a little four-year-old boy on the ward who was dying of malnourishment. Prone and still, hooked up to an IV, his little stomach protruding, the only sign of life he exhibited was his shallow, intermittent breathing. His mother, a mere skeleton of a woman herself, was curled up beside her baby son, sleeping from exhaustion. When the pediatric team awoke her in the morning, she sat up with an embarrassed start, fixing her sari, and staring demurely down at the floor. She didn't, however, remove a protective arm from over her son.

"What is this? Why haven't you been feeding the boy properly?" the attending physician barked out.

The woman didn't reply, but continued staring at the floor like a guilty child.

The doctor went on to talk above the mother's head about the specifics of the child's management. When he was done, he stared at her scornfully.

"Like a bunch of animals. How can they have babies when they can't even care for them?" he muttered, before walking away.

And then she looked up. I can't forget the sight of those enormous tear-filled eyes that swallowed up the woman's taut-skinned, bony face. I wouldn't be surprised if she had kept her son alive this long by giving up her own food. I wondered when she had eaten her last meal. When she caught my eye, however, she ducked her head remorsefully down again. There wasn't a trace of anger about her, only abject acceptance of our medical team's condemnation.

My time in both Delhi and Calcutta opened my eyes to the true luxury in which I am able to practice medicine in the U.S. With ample supplies of medical necessities, such as needles, gloves, and blood—and far fewer medical headaches, such as black-market needle sellers, cockroaches, and aggressive monkeys—very few American medical professionals can even imagine what it might be like to practice medicine in a less advantageous setting. I at least have been granted a glimpse into that different reality.

I have also grown to realize that my fantasy of practicing medicine in a developing country is not an easy one to come by. Indeed, the experience of rotating through India is perhaps best described through the story of my friend Jen, an American medical student I met during my tenure at AIIMS. Like many of us, Jen was extremely idealistic about going to an impoverished country and contributing her services. India taught her, however, that "help" is a relative word. When she first arrived, for instance, to live in a dormitory near the hospital, she found that she was to share her room with some interesting mates—families of cockroaches, ants, and other unidentifiable flying, crawling, and stinging creepie-crawlies. Not only was she harassed by these intruders in her home, but whenever she, a light-haired white woman, went out on the street alone, she was harassed by groups of boys who whistled, commented, bumped into, pinched, and pried at her. And then, there was the infamous Dr. Singh, who, upon seeing her improperly stamped papers, actually threw them at her face, shouting, "Get out of my sight!" By the time she set up another rotation and managed to feel comfortable traveling around New Delhi by herself, she encountered something even worse. On her way home from the hospital in one of Delhi's characteristic little motor-scooter-pulled rickshaws, two thugs jumped into the open vehicle on either side of her, scaring her out of her wits, and making off with her bag, in which were not only her medical equipment, but her travelers checks and her tickets home. To add insult to injury, she was barely recovering from these harrowing adventures when, at a picnic, she and another American woman were accosted by a group of New Delhi thugs worse than insects, muggers, and rude physicians combined—monkeys. Poor Jen actually had a monkey leap upon her shoulders, pull her hair, and make off with her lunch-filled cloth satchel. And yet, after all this, she ended up having a wonderful time in India. I remember sitting in front of the majestic Taj Mahal with her when she turned to me and said, "So when are we doing this again?"

India is not an easy country to love. But when you get past the craziness, the contradictions, the heat, and the inconvenience, you find something rare, and stirring, and real. It shocks you down to your toes, only to fill you up again with wonder—not unlike (and I say this grudgingly) training to be a physician. I guess if someone like Jen can learn to love India, I could learn to at least like medicine.

My time as a medical student in India was vital in defining my adult cultural self. Not as a schizophrenic now-Indian, now-American, but as an integrated person who is both Indian and American simultaneously, in all settings, and with confidence. Ultimately, I grew to realize that my professional selfhood, my competence, and my mobility are not antithetical to being an Indian woman. Rather, they are traits that I can utilize to define and assert that cultural identity.

My disguise, already burdensome during Indian vacations, grew stifling to the point of strangulation during these two excursions. As the land of India herself is contradictory and difficult, but rewarding, so, too, my complicated selfhood is a burden I cannot shirk in any cultural setting. And like that country that has historically integrated rather than forgotten, layered rather than obliterated, and ultimately colonized even her colonizers, I, too, am simultaneously my many selves—doctor, writer, Indian chick. It's a jostling, often pothole-ridden journey, avoiding obstacles of both man and beast, but it's my journey, and at least I'm learning something on the way. If my back were decorated by vehicle-art, I think it might be an image of a bindi-ed, stethoscoped, jeans-clad physician, with the creatively spelled caption, "Laydee Daktaar on Bored."

To OB? Or Not to OB?

I may not be the prince of Denmark. I may not be haunted by the ghost of my dead father. (Daddy's hale and hearty, thank you.) I may not bear any resemblance whatsoever to Sir Laurence Olivier or even Kenneth Branaugh. But I have stared, bleary-eyed, into the eerie face of a skull (Ah, my cadaver, I knew him well), and I have, for the majority of my fourth year of medical school, been tortured by the existential question, "To be or not to be?" Or, in my case, to OB or not to OB?

The fourth year is the best time of medical school. Or so they say. After completing two rigorous years of classroom basic science, followed by a hectic year of required clinical rotations, the fourth year is supposed to be a time of electives, relaxation, and residency planning. It is a time to look forward to what all of medical training prepares one for: to be a doctor in the field of one's choosing. The problem for me, like Hamlet, was in the choosing.

I came to medical school to do OB/Gyn. This predisposition was undoubtedly inspired by the same forces that pushed me into medicine. Having no physicians in my family, my medical role models were all television inspired. Although I loved Hawkeye and all the guys on *St.*

Elsewhere, there didn't seem any real place for me in either type of "front lines." But then I saw my first female physician role model from the tube: a dynamic woman OB/Gyn running her own holistic women's health center. I knew then that I, too, wanted to run my own holistic health center, replete with not only a bevy of women's services, including health care, counseling, and a legal clinic, but also child care, a community meeting space, and outreach facilities. By the time I got to college, the fantasy had grown more elaborate, and I had added a music room, art gallery, bookstore, and café to my women's clinic fantasy. (Because, as every good college student knows, there is no harm in being a holistic clinic doc and general do-gooder while simultaneously being well-read and over caffeinated as well.) Like my oh-so-realistic role model from TV I planned to practice wonderful medicine, deliver delightful babies, have a passionate relationship, play on the beach with my golden retriever, and look great doing it all. It was only when I came to medical school that I realized television was merely a stage, and the good doctor merely a player.

OB/Gyn is no walk, or even jog, on the beach. None of medicine is, in fact. But OB/Gyn, the field of my budding feminist fantasies, the field that any lay person would assume to be the most woman-friendly and nurturant, is not in the least way holistic, warm, or even always pro-woman. I'm not saying that all OB/Gyn physicians are terrible (in fact, the one physician I have grown to admire the most at Hopkins is an amazing, dynamic OB/Gyn working with HIV-positive women). It is just that the field is a predominantly surgical one, and with that reality comes a rush-rush, overworked, and not in the least fuzzy-wuzzy culture. It is a field that too often hardens its residents, robbing

them of sleep, a personal life, and any semblance of pre-
dictability. (Babies, emergency C-sections, and massive
vaginal bleeding are hardly events that stick to schedule.)
But with all that—I loved it. Well, most of it. I loved deliv-
ering babies (I cried almost every time), I loved diag-
nosing and treating STDs (even the really yucky ones),
and I especially loved being in clinic with well women (I
felt like a true women's advocate, my heart on my sleeve,
her legs in the air, the speculum in my hands). I just didn't
love being in the operating room. I've never been much
of a seamstress, you can't chat up a sleeping patient, and
during long cases, all I could think about was how much
my feet hurt. But, I figured, I could learn to live with that.

It was just that my life was already so complicated. By
the end of my third year of medical school my writing
career was already taking off, I had found the man I
wanted to spend the rest of my life with, and I was coming to realize, more and more, that the hierarchy and
strict obeisance that medicine demanded was not suited
to my independent spirit. And so, I did a rather Hamlet-
like thing. I ran away. In between my third and fourth
years of medical school, I did an eleven-month Masters
of Public Health (MPH) program at the Johns Hopkins
School of Hygiene and Public Health.

Wolfe Street is the widest road in America, or so the
saying goes. And as Wolfe is the street that divides Johns
Hopkins hospital from the Public Health school, there is
a good degree of truth behind that statement. My year at
the Public Health school was diametrically opposite to
my previous experiences across Wolfe Street. International, accomplished students who rivaled only the faculty in the diversity of their interests and experiences
studied together in an atmosphere I found challenging,

thrilling, and incredibly warm. I met physicians who had dodged bullets in Bosnia, family planning advocates who conducted condom campaigns throughout remote Pakistan, and environmental engineers who precisely calculated the relative risk between drinking a glass of tap water in Rio de Janeiro and Baltimore. I worked incredibly hard. But I woke up happy every day. No one expected me to hide my creative instincts, no one expected me to conform to any rigid or hierarchical cultural standard, and certainly, no one asked me questions about obscure biochemical pathways in between asking me to pick up jelly donuts for the team and put in the new patient's Foley catheter. Being away from medical school and the hospital, I realized a few fundamental truths about myself: I loved public health; I loved writing; I loved working in a warm, international, academic environment (with colleagues who would just as heartily address issues of global concern as go salsa dancing); I loved my intellectual freedom; I loved my personal life.

Coming back to medical school was hard. Facing my residency decision, albeit a year later than most of my former classmates, was even harder. I was in existential agony, and awoke, night after night, in cold sweats, haunted by ghosts of my own making. I had come to medical school to pursue a career in women's health. I truly enjoyed most aspects of OB/Gyn. It fit my politics. It fit many of my professional goals. It was just too all-consuming to allow any time, energy, or room for much else—professionally or personally. I could see no way but to drop out of medicine altogether.

And then came a compromise. And it came in the form of a teenage girl. Not any one girl in particular, of course, but the entire cohort of pimply, moody, and hor-

monally overcharged women-to-be. As Hamlet's quest
led him away from his true love, mine led me straight
to that flowery-haired, dreamy-eyed personification of
childhood-womanhood, Ophelia. While Ophelia may
not at first consideration seem the ideal symbol of her
modern counterparts—she is a dead literary character
whose discovery of her sexuality lead to insanity, not
teen motherhood, illicit drugs, or STDs—let's just consider her the representative of her beleaguered age
group. And as that, what she represents to me is hope: a
career solution that does not require that my personal
life and sanity drown in the abyss of professional demands. Adolescent medicine gives me the opportunity
to work with young people, still dealing with gynecologi-
cal issues, infectious diseases, reproduction, and STDs,
but from a more community-based, family-oriented, and
ultimately, nonsurgical vantage point. It is furthermore a
career decision I can live with, combining writing with
practice, clinical work with public health, policy making
with child rearing.

For this decision, I have been not only haunted by the
ghost of my once potential career, but by the very real
goblins who are my colleagues and teachers. "I really
hate people who sell themselves short, talking about
family life and all that," one classmate had unexpectedly
reprimanded me upon hearing my last-minute career
switch. "I mean, you are in control of your own destiny,
you know. You can't wimp out like that."

And that was the idea, that choosing family life, that
choosing pediatrics, for that matter, was essentially
"wimping out." I was a soldier gone AWOL, a weak marine, a deviant not marching to the hard-core drummer.

Regardless, after much rumination and writing (not to

mention a few bouts of self-indulgent weeping—I'm
sure even Hamlet indulged in a good cry now and again),
I have come to the realization that medicine, for me,
must ultimately be about compromise. There are no perfect solutions, only approximate ones. There is no answer
to the existential question, only some good guesses. Ultimately, I cannot be paralyzed into bitter inaction merely
because I don't like the system. I have decided not to
suffer the slings and arrows of medicine's outrageous
fortune, but to make my own. I have decided it is nobler
not to OB, but just be.

THE BIG TRANSITION

0_2

There are a lot of ways to deliver life's breath, and not all of them are medical.

Of the latter, the names are scientific and decidedly un-poetic: Nasal cannula, blowby, facemask, and continuous positive airway pressure (CPAP), to name a few. If you want to get fancy and add some machines that not only deliver oxygen, but do the work for you, you would add to the list conventional ventilators as well as the more exotic jet and high frequency oscillators that shake, rattle, and roll you even as they keep you alive.

But that's just a lot of esoteric words if you don't know what they mean. Like most of medicine.

The bottom line—the simple, pure fact of the matter—is we all need something to keep us going. In and out, over and over, we all need to breathe.

My transition from medical school to internship has not been an easy one. Not only was I graduating from school and beginning a frightening new job, but I had to find a new apartment, move to a new city, finish a book project, and, most overwhelming of all, get married. My wedding, an intercultural Indo-Teutonic affair set in the heart of New Jersey, was brilliantly planned a mere three days before I was to graduate medical school and a mere six weeks before I was to begin internship. It was a joyous time, but the stress of my impending internship added a heightened sense of panic to what was in and of itself a pretty big life event. By the time I got married, gallivanted around the Iberian Peninsula on a whirlwind honeymoon, packed, moved, and finished orientation, I was exhausted.

"I could sleep for a month," I told my mother.

"I could sleep for a year," I told my new husband.

"I could sleep forever," I told the shrink.

And it still wasn't even July 1.

I've never done transitions well. I could never sleep the night before the first day of school. As I grew older, I raised pre-finals jitters to new heights. So a wedding, move, graduation, and internship were enough to send me into the worst panic of my life.

You remember the scene in *The Graduate* where Dustin Hoffman sits at the bottom of the pool with his scuba gear on? He can see everyone through the refractive filter of the water—they're moving their arms, eating barbecue, having fun—but he can't interact with them, or even hear them. His ears are plugged—by a combination of the water, scuba equipment, and Simon and Garfunkel soundtrack.

That's how I felt as I began my internship. It was all— glub, glub—bottom of the pool oppressive drowny feelings. And I didn't even have an O_2 tank with me.

An internship sucks any way you cut it. It's a lot of hours, a lot of hard work, and a lot of energy that doesn't leave much reserved for anything else. Sleeping and eating become prized, rare events that are cherished with a fervor only previously lent to worn-out comfort blankies of childhood. It's an initiation, just like medical school, but somehow, more intense. The stress of four years packaged into one yearlong sleepless night. Perhaps I exaggerate. To hear it from my medical school professors, we in the modern age have it easy. During their prehistoric internships, those days when they had to walk to the hospital uphill both ways, barefoot through the year-round snow—they worked longer, harder hours, drew all their own bloods and analyzed them too, shot and developed their own X-rays, and only visited their families upon express permission from their attendings. I guess, exaggeration aside, it was pretty tough back then. I guess the benefits made the excesses of training worth it. I guess people were just willing to put up with more crap. But in the modern age of managed care medical salaries and unemployed M.D.s, it's becoming a little ridiculous. But still, for people who really want to be doctors that badly, I guess it's still worth it. For me, the problem is, I just don't want it that badly.

Hee Hee Hee—Hah.

Hee Hee Hee—Hah.

Lamaze breathing. The rhythmic quality is supposed to help a woman through labor. Why is it only reserved for reproductive and not productive labor? I too need something to help me breathe.

There is a pressure on my chest and a burning in my eyes and a crawling on my skin and a gurgling in my stomach, and I am thinking, this can't be normal, this can't be normal, this can't be normal.

On my honeymoon, my honeymoon, for God's sake, I was throwing up because I was so freaked-out. So freaked. So scared. I couldn't enjoy this new life I was starting because I knew that it would soon be snatched out of my hands.

A woman, no matter how overeducated, should at least be given the liberty to enjoy her honeymoon.

Six hours behind. America is six hours behind us. I would calculate this fact every day with my husband. We would have this conversation over *café con leche* at an adorable little sidewalk restaurant we would visit before our daily pilgrimage to the Mediterranean. I will call the dean this evening. I will call the program at five. I will call my parents after it's all said and done.

Go for it, go for it, he would say, but I could see the unease in his eyes. What would I do instead? He did not ask. What will I do instead? I asked for him. I'll support you, baby, I'll support you, baby, I'll support you, baby, he would say. But our debt? Our bills? Our rent?

We would leave the questions unanswered and spend our evenings drinking wine at out-of-the-way mountain inns.

In Madrid, after a late-night flamenco show, the owner of the taverna actually offered me a job. When I explained, but I'm not a dancer, I'm not even Spanish, she said it didn't matter. I had the right look and she would teach me, she said, she would teach me. With my dark hair and eyes and dramatic face, she could teach me to be a flamenco dancer.

I almost took her up on it.

The moment we landed in Dulles airport, I called the dean of my medical school. From the airport. Right there with my luggage piled all around me and my honeymoon tan not even faded a little bit yet, I called. I was filled with the Iberian sun and Mediterranean wine and offers of flamenco-dancing careers and they had made me brave enough to turn away from this life I had hated for so long, this life that made me so unhappy, this life that everyone expected me to live but myself. He wasn't available to talk to me, but I cried on the phone to his secretary.

The next day we met, and he zapped the sun right out of me. He silenced the sounds of the clicking castanets that were playing in my ears. It wouldn't be wise, he said. Not wise at all. And overachieving me had never done anything unwise.

"Are you sure, Sayantani," he said, "that you never want to practice clinical medicine again?"

I wasn't.

If I quit, he said, that was what I would basically be guaranteeing, and after all my hard work I wouldn't want to close any doors permanently, would I?

I wouldn't.

Glub, glub. And there I was again, at the bottom of the pool, watching everyone else eating barbecue.

Moving. To our cute new apartment in Westchester. Oh how I wanted just to be a new wife and cook on our brand spanking new indoor grill (salmon and peppers and little *croup de etes*). Oh how I wanted to decorate and pick china settings and dress pretty and smell good. Oh how I wanted to enjoy, just a little, this amazing new life I was beginning.

But there it was. A smelly new hospital. And new people I didn't know. And patients. And responsibilities. And everyone calling me Doctor.

Who, me?

I went to see one of the administrative heads of my new program. An amazing, gentle woman who made me feel both better and worse.

"I was depressed too, very seriously, after the birth of my child," she told me.

I guess that meant she thought I was depressed. I wasn't sure she was right, but oh, how her sympathy felt good and oh, how it felt comforting to have a label that I could just crouch under. And what if I was depressed? That wasn't a crime. Plenty of people got depressed and here was this nice motherly woman telling me it was OK and they would give me time off if I needed it and they would look into disability payments and all of this stuff.

But then I went to see the psychiatrist, and he laughed at my self-deprecating jokes and he appreciated my wit even in my blues and he said to me, "You don't seem depressed to me. You just seem like you don't want to be a doctor."

And I'm afraid he was right.

It's not that I don't want to be a doctor per se. If I was already a fully trained doctor, for instance, I would be perfectly happy to do child advocacy and health communications and public health and write policy and influence governments and set up programs. I just don't want to get all of this agonizing clinical training if it's not what I want to do anyway.

"I have this fire in me," I told the shrink in one of those moments of articulate insight I tend to get when spilling my guts, "and it's to write. I just don't know how much longer I can hold on to it. This medicine thing is killing my fire. And soon, there won't be even a spark."

Dramatic stuff, but true.

He seemed inspired. Maybe he was a frustrated writer too. But that didn't stop him from writing me a prescription for sleeping pills. He offered me some Valium too, but I didn't take him up on the offer.

"Lots of residents get reactive depression," he said in

his loud, jovial voice, "and most of them do fine. Sometimes a little benzodiazepine is just the trick to take the edge off." He patted me paternally on my back. "Sometimes I don't wonder if all doctors don't need a little downer now and again."

After the shrink, I call my agent. To ask for leads. To ask for advice.

"Are you kidding?" she asks. "Do you want to lose your book contract?"

"No, of course not." I am confused. What does one have to do with another?

"You're writing a book about medicine. And how is your publisher supposed to market you if you're a dropout?" She pauses.

"I have a lot of degrees," I begin.

"That's really no guarantee of anything," she says. "Welcome to the real world."

Hee Hee Hee—Hah.

Hee Hee Hee—Hah.

After the agent, my last stop is another professor—this time, the head of my particular program, the man who had interviewed me, the man who had influenced me to come to this little-heard-of program in the godforsaken Bronx. His smile reminds me of the Mediterranean sun and all those *café con leches*.

We talk about Joseph Campbell. Finding your bliss and all that. I am pretty sure that medicine is *not* my bliss but he says, I don't think you're the kind of writer that wants to lock herself up in an Ivory Tower like Emily Dickinson. I see you as a Toni Morrison, as an activist and a writer, as a mover and a shaker, as a leader and a worker and a doctor and everything.

He saw in me his mentor, he said, a woman who had

worn silver bangles and hid Guatemalan refugees in her basement and driven a too-fast red sports car even though she preached about the bourgeoisie and raged against the institutions of oppression. Her husband, he added in an amusing side note, was also white, like mine, but he was even more white than Boris because he was actually English, and a literature professor at that, and he sported a long, thin ponytail, which as we all know, is the most telltale sign of white-itude. And this bangle-wearing, sports-car driving, Guatemalan-hiding mentor of his actually reminded him of me.

And worse still, this beautiful, passionate doctor had died a young, untimely death after battling nobly and long and uncomplainingly.

How could I fight that many metaphors? And a dead, beautiful mentor besides? How could I complain when I wasn't even dying and didn't even have a green-card holder in my apartment?

I smiled and thanked him and agreed. No, I didn't want to be like Emily and yes I did want to be like Toni and oh, finding your bliss is hard and yes, I was willing to go the distance because my dream was that red-hot. But the sunshine he gave me lasted only so long. By the time I got home I was already cold.

The air was so thin. I had to strain to get enough oxygen.

My first rotation is fortuitous—the nursery, which combines my interests in OB/Gyn and pediatrics. All I do is run to deliveries on the labor floor to resuscitate little tykes who are blue, or drugged, or too, too young to live without complicated technologies. One of the main things we do is give them oxygen (blowby, facemask) because, as we explain to the anxious daddies who peer over at us, it helps them get used to breathing in the real world rather than breathing inside mommy's tummy. (Pediatricians, I learn, like to use words like mommy and tummy. It's hard to avoid the habit and I start to say those things too.)

I hold a little tube blowing air over their little faces until they turn the right color (pink, not blue) and start crying normally (we don't, however, turn them upside down and spank them under any circumstances), and look generally like they're going to make the difficult transition from dark and cozy to bright and cold and harsh. When they're feeling better, they tend to reach out and grab the oxygen catheter and crookedly hold it up to their faces, like some little performance microphone. A first solo. It's pretty damn adorable.

There's actually something called "the tongue sign," I learn. That's when you know a baby is really going to be OK. That's when, after stressful moments of blue lips and limp bodies and low heartbeats, a baby gets it together and decides to take the plunge into life in this crazy outside world. Bit by bit, so subtly that you don't even notice it at first, the baby will slither out its little, juicy, pink, newborn tongue in an eyes-closed, what-the-heck-is-that-new-stimulus gesture.

They're tasting the oxygen. And I guess it tastes pretty good.

I too am trying, crying, struggling, and wondering when I'll turn from blue to pink. I rage, and wail, and stick out my tongue, and try to taste what this new life is to be like.

I'm still not so sure.

Help, help, I am calling. Help. But no one notices. They can't hear me. They're all busy above the water, laughing, joking, eating barbecue. Glub, glub. I leave watermarks all over my new manuscript.

The Gender Wars

Models, Mentors, and Motherhood: Raising Future Female Physicians

"We welcome women in surgery." The statement seemed to resound for a moment in the green sterility of the O.R. The scrub nurse paused in her countings and recountings of lap sponges, while the drowsy anesthesiologist awoke to peer curiously from behind his curtain. I, the third-year medical student precariously poised in order to grasp and pull retractors, was so startled I almost dropped my cramped body into the sterile field. It was six weeks into my basic surgical rotation, and I had seen very little if any sign of welcome. Long hours, sexually charged jokes, and the verbal tyranny of hot-tempered prima donna surgeons had not impressed upon me the idea that surgery was particularly woman friendly. And yet, here was this hotshot attending surgeon informing me to the contrary. Then the other shoe fell.

"Yeah, we welcome women," he sniggered, "we welcome women in surgery because they open up more job opportunities for men." Thinking that his sophisticated comments needed clarification, he added, "because women don't stay on in the workplace, you know."

I tried to keep my eyes neutral above my mask. They ached to shoot daggers.

Then came the banal analysis. "Despite the feminist

movement," he explained, "women are still basically mothers at heart. It's instinct. And you can't fight instinct."

That's when my eyes started to sting. Perhaps it was from all the daggers I never let myself shoot in med school, when I had listened passively to equally offensive remarks, and not allowed myself to speak. I thought of all the women in my family who had struggled so that I could get where I was now. The surgeon's callousness and my own inability to protest put me on the brink of losing self-control. Then something interesting happened. The scrub nurse, a middle-aged African American woman, took the moment when my eyes were most wet to bump me lightly. "Sorry, baby," she drawled smoothly, locking her warm brown eyes with mine, "for bumpin' into you." Her eyes glowed with strength and understanding. "You all right?"

I wish there was a woman physician I could have turned to after that particular incident in the O.R. As with many other times, I could have desperately used the support of an older woman already established in the field. And yet, although I have come into contact with women physicians during most of my basic science classes and all my clinical rotations, there is no woman I can call my very own "mentor." The same formal distance that exists between most of my male instructors and myself is quite evident with female instructors as well.

"Medicine will make a man out of anyone." This poignant phrase, which holds more symbolic significance than literal truth, has been proven real for me throughout my years at medical school. Despite the increasing female presence in the profession of medicine, the culture of medicine remains male-dominated, and the field tries to mold all of us in its image. For instance, in the hallowed halls of Hopkins internal medicine, the residents are called Osler marines, are required to wear their Hopkins insignia-patterned "Osler ties" every Friday, and are censured when they don't do their work the "Oslerian way." Indeed, when rotating through internal medicine, I was told by one attending physician that medicine was like religion at Johns Hopkins, and that going to Grand Rounds was like going to church. These rituals are so blatantly patriarchal they are surreal. Indeed, they remind me of my college friend Mona, whose elder brother would use her for his childhood target practice, yelling, "Be a man, Mona, be a man," while he whirled baseballs at her head. This misbegotten, though well-intentioned, attempt to "toughen" Mona up is very much like the molding of women in medicine. But while we are pelted with the baseballs of male medical tradition, where are our female mentors?

While I had an abundance of female mentors in college, I have strongly felt a lack of female physician mentoring in med school. Perhaps this is because medicine has "made a man" out of mentoring. By this, I mean that within the culture of medicine, the very nature of mentoring, like the nature of being a good doctor, remains patriarchally defined. Just as the model of being a "good physician" is a male one (i.e., valuing qualities such as aggressiveness, hierarchy, working long hours, putting career ahead of family, etc.), the model of mentorship within medicine is also made for and by men. Thus, the pattern of mentorship I have witnessed in med school is heavily steeped in hierarchy, discipline, distance, and respect. Although it is possible for women to mentor in this pattern, it is, for me, an unnatural, unfamiliar, and unwanted model of relationship. Indeed, the pattern of mentoring I feel most familiar with is one of emotional closeness rather than hierarchy and distance.

My mother, an activist, professor, and writer, has been my strongest mentor. Indeed, while Western cultures often diminish the power of maternal mentoring, my immigrant parents' Indian culture has instilled in me a great respect for the strength of motherhood. Bengal, the region of India where my parents hail from, is perhaps one of the only cultures left where goddess-worshiping is still the norm, and mothers, earthly embodiments of the great goddesses, are considered to have awesome power. It is this more maternal ideal of mentorship, which involves encouragement and challenge as well as comfort and care, that I find most effective in my life.

Interestingly enough, I have found such a pattern of mentorship in med school. However, these "maternal mentors" are not physicians. They are the nurses, physicians' assistants, secretaries, and housekeepers who create an almost underground network of female support within the hospital. This invisible net has caught me time and time again. For example, during my OB/Gyn clerkship, a scrub nurse I called "Miss Rosa" invariably had my size gloves out before even the attending physicians'. She made room for me at the O.R. table, shoving me forward, suction scissors or retractor in hand. It was she, not the residents or the attendings, who made sure I was able to attend each and every interesting case. "Paging Dr. Say, paging Dr. Say," she would call down the hallway. "Come on, Baby Doc, there's a case goin' in right now. Ain't you gonna operate?" Within the oftentimes hostile environment of medical school, it is these small encouragements that keep me going.

Early in my second year, I heard a talk given by a dynamic female orthopedic surgeon. She described how, as the sole woman in her residency program, she was given a locker in the nurses' locker room. In order to fight the isolation, she apparently stormed into the men's locker room one day, and to the chagrin of her colleagues, proceeded to change in there from that day forth. At the end of her speech, when I went up to talk to her, she briskly handed me her card, saying, "I'm very interested in mentoring female medical students. Call me sometime." Although I continue to have great admiration for this physician, I never did call her. Quite frankly, she made me nervous. I'm not sure I had enough medically savvy things to speak to her about. While my network of maternal mentors support me through chitchats about family, romance, and hospital politics, I feel like my relationships with women physicians must necessarily be about medicine. There is no room to slack, to doubt, to question, to fear.

Undoubtedly, older women physicians have had to fight hard to break into the male locker room. However, I don't see the point of subsuming myself into someone else's model, nor do I think it is wise to distance ourselves from our nonphysician sources of female support—the nurses and others in the women's locker room. Both the culture of medicine and the culture of mentoring must be true to who we are—as women, as physicians. It's time to get out of the male locker room and make a room of our own.

In the Company of Women

In the years when all the other little girls had pictures of Shaun Cassidy, Davy Jones, or a rainbow-horned unicorn on their walls, my bedroom landscape was quite different. As the daughter of a 1970s women's activist, it was the faces of the Great White Feminist Foremothers—Elizabeth Cady Stanton, Susan B. Anthony, Elizabeth Blackwell—who stared down at me every night of my childhood. I remember feeling simultaneously inspired by and unconnected to these large-hatted, dour-faced women. They didn't look particularly friendly. Later, I learned to look up to women of color as well as those mainstream feminists. When I eventually found myself entering Dr. Blackwell's profession, however, I couldn't help but remember that childhood poster.

Shortly after Elizabeth Blackwell enrolled as the first woman student at Geneva Medical College in 1847, many all-female medical schools were born in the U.S. The women who attended these institutions have been described by historians as "united by their critique of male physicians and the medicine they were practicing on women patients."[15] These women physicians, suppos-

[15] E. B. Thomas, "How Women Medical Students First Came to Johns Hopkins," 38–45.

edly, intended to apply "feminine" qualities—such as nurturing and empathy for women—to medical fields such as pediatrics, obstetrics, and gynecology. Women who attended these schools were different, undoubtedly, from women who chose to attend predominantly male institutions such as Johns Hopkins. Indeed, accounts of three of Johns Hopkins pioneering women—Dorothy Reed, Florence Sabin, and Margaret Long—show that these women had quite a different outlook. These three women went on to do great things. Reed was a pathologist after whom the Reed-Sternberg cell (pathognomonic of Hodgkin's disease) is named; Sabin was a prominent physician-scientist and the first female member of the National Academy of Sciences; and Long was a tuberculosis researcher who played a prominent role in the establishment of tuberculosis sanitoriums in the '40s and '50s. But regardless of what they did later, they were all Johns Hopkins medical students, and among some of the earliest classes at the coeducational institution.[16]

When I was applying to medical school, I interviewed at a number of different places. While I didn't have the option of an all-women's medical school, I did visit schools that differed widely in their culture, tone, and history. Although Johns Hopkins was, by reputation, one of the most conservative and traditional schools around, the people I met during my interview day convinced me that the place had changed. Hopkins was now interested in the arts and sciences, in the humanities, and in healing rather than just in medicine, they told me. The Old Boy tradition of the past was no more; Johns

[16] Shrager, "Three Women at Johns Hopkins," 56–69.

Hopkins was gearing up for a new era of public health and liberalism. And so, over other medical schools with more progressive reputations, I chose to go to Hopkins.

Drs. Reed, Sabin, and Long probably knew that there would be a distinct difference between Hopkins and any all-women's medical institution. And yet they chose to attend a coeducational school during the late nineteenth century. Joseph B. Shrager, a surgeon from the University of Pennsylvania, writes about their motivation for doing so, their coping mechanisms, and their experiences while at Hopkins. Reading this account, I was impressed by the similarities and differences of these early physicians' years at Hopkins with mine.

Shrager asks an interesting question: whether these early Hopkins women were proponents of a "feminine medicine," or if they were simply female physicians. To begin with, he looks at their motivation for entering medicine. Like their modern counterparts, the reasons that Reed, Sabin, and Long entered medicine ranged from the philanthropic to the more avaricious. While Reed wrote in her journal that her "plans" were to "try and do some work . . . which would help mankind" and her "pleasures" were "helping others,"[17] it was also true that both Sabin and Reed needed to contribute financially to their families. Ultimately, however, none of these three women expressed any larger commitment to the feminist medical movement, and in Shrager's opinion, all three of them defined themselves first as physicians, second as women physicians. Reed, for instance, was critical in her journal of politicized or feminist medical students. She described one female classmate as "super-

[17] Ibid., 565.

sensitive, looking for discrimination and slights" and another as typifying "the freak woman in medicine—that all the rest of us normal students could not live down."[18]

A century later, the same schism between women in medicine remains. Although I, for instance, went to medical school because I saw medicine as a concrete tool to affect social change, few of my classmates were that politicized in their motivations. At the most, many admitted to philanthropic rationale, while some openly admitted that they were in medicine for the prestige or the money. In regard to political organizations, therefore, there were far fewer at Hopkins than I had seen during my undergraduate days. There were only a couple of feminist organizations in my medical school, including chapters of The American Medical Women's Association (AMWA) and Medical Students for Choice. I call them feminist organizations, but I suspect that there would be some argument with me on that score. Indeed, the anti-feminist backlash that afflicts many women of my generation disproportionately affects women in medical school. While the handful of progressive organizations at Hopkins were patronized by a small number of students, it was only a fraction of that already tiny group who would feel comfortable with the word feminism.

I have always been fairly political. As a teenager and college student, I joined a number of feminist groups, and was a vocal participant in many progressive organizations. Therefore, I was very enthusiastic at the prospect of forming liberal alliances in medical school. At my first AMWA meeting, however, I noticed a strange dynamic. I was the only woman of color in the room. Indeed, as I

[18] Ibid.

was to soon realize, many of the African American women
in the class were involved in the minority medical students'
association (SNMA), which was understandably preoccupied with issues of racism and diversity. As with many
women of color, they were forced by the conservative, Old
Boy environment of Hopkins to prioritize their oppres-
sions; and as usual, race was ranked higher than gender. I
found myself in a difficult position due to these political
schisms. While I would have naturally aligned myself with
the people of color, they quite blatantly did not include me.
Indeed, to my shock, the minority students' organization at
Hopkins does not recognize Asian Americans as minori-
ties for the ostensible reason that Asian Americans are not
a minority by number in the medical profession. I find that
ridiculous, since we are most definitely a racial and ethnic
minority in this country and deserve to have our oppression recognized. In addition, excluding us from minority
organizations only reinforces the stereotype of Asian
Americans as the upwardly mobile, problem-free, apoliti-
cal "model minority," and widens the already existing gaps
between us and other people of color.

So I tried to bridge the gap. Since the minority organization didn't recognize my experience or my oppression,
I hoped to diversify the feminist group. Yet when I
brought this issue of diversity up at meetings, it met only
a lukewarm response. "Should we have a potluck and in-
vite the women of color?" one woman asked. I tried not
to cringe at their tokenistic attitude. "Why don't you
take charge of including more of the women of color,
Sayantani?" another requested. What did that make me,
I thought, the diversity fairy?

It was the same thing I had heard from my mother's
mainstream feminist colleagues in the 1970s. Although

women were ostensibly concerned over the lack of diversity in their groups, they weren't willing to question themselves, and wonder what they were doing to make women of color feel unwelcome. Similarly, my colleagues couldn't understand why women of different backgrounds, different cultures—both ethnic and socio-economic—and different agendas weren't flocking to their meetings. And after a few halfhearted attempts at inclusion, they didn't really bother.

These women were the liberal ones. The rest of my class was filled with women who were fairly complacent and satisfied with the gender status quo. They probably didn't differ too much from that early female physician, Dorothy Reed, who considered feminists "supersensitive freaks." After one sexist lecture, I remember, when a surgeon repeatedly emphasized the importance of doing low abdominal incisions on women since "all they really care about is looking good in their bikinis," a group of the more progressive women in my class decided to formally protest. We received an enormous amount of flak from some other women in the class, who felt we were being "oversensitive" and "overreacting."

It's interesting to note that physicians' sexist senses of humor have not changed that much in a century. Dorothy Reed writes about a lecture on nasal disorders that she and Margaret Long attended, where the speaker, pointedly directing his comments at the two women, compared, for the greater part of his lecture, the nasal passages to the corpus spongiosa of the penis. Although Reed "cried all the way home—hysterically" and Long "swore," they were happy enough to dismiss the incident from their minds. Some "heartfelt apologies" from fellow students were enough to convince Reed that "all was right with the world."[19] If she had been a modern woman, she might have been among my classmates who thought we were making too much of a simple joke, essentially upbraiding our rocking of the proverbial boat. Indeed, despite her distress at that nasal-penile incident, Reed soon afterward vowed to "accept any treatment as long as it was the same as would be applied to a man." She further wrote in her journal that she would "ask no favors because of being a woman." As Shrager writes, she wanted to "do all in her power to be accepted on men's terms in a man's world."[20]

I have heard it said that women, on the average, enter medical school with higher scores than their male colleagues, but leave with significantly lower ones. Undoubtedly this phenomenon, if true, arises from the fact that women have to succeed in an environment that is often both overtly and covertly hostile to them. While two of the three women discussed in Shrager's article graduated ranked number two and four from their medical school class, all of the women remarked on the pervasive sexism throughout their medical training. On her first day in Baltimore in 1896, for instance, Reed took a carriage ride to the Hopkins medical campus. Beside her sat a gentleman who "crudely and arrogantly stud(ied) her physique from head to toe." When she alighted from the carriage in front of the medical school, he asked her if she was entering. When she said yes, he replied, "Don't. Go home," and proceeded into the administrative building. Reed was to later discover that this rude man was none other than Hopkins's famous William Osler—the first chairman of medicine

[19] Ibid., 566.
[20] Ibid.

who is to this day revered. Four years later, when Reed and Sabin's high academic standings gave them the opportunity to fill two of four prestigious internships under Osler, they would be harangued and badgered by their classmates to give up their spots. When they did not, an attending physician suggested to Reed that the only reason she was willing to take the internship, and accept the accompanying responsibility of the black male wards, was "to satisfy her abnormal sexual curiosity."[21]

Institutional sexism has, over the last hundred years, gained some degree of sophistication. It is, however, still alive and well at Hopkins. In the times of our physician foremothers, for instance, menstruation was considered a stumbling block to women's work and education.[22] At the end of the twentieth century, we have not progressed much beyond that. Family life and future parental responsibilities, real concerns for all physicians, are too often the barriers to women's medical careers. When advising my husband, then fiancé, and me about residency decisions, for instance, a top Hopkins administrator was much more preoccupied with Boris's decision than mine. He was deeply concerned about Boris getting into the most competitive radiation oncology program possible, while his attitude to me was one of indulgent support. "You'll be able to take time off to raise a family," he commented after hearing that I had resolved to go into pediatrics rather than OB/Gyn. "It will be a less rigorous field." While family life was one of the factors in my residency decision, it wasn't something I had mentioned to this administrator. Although motherhood

[21] Ibid.
[22] Ibid.

is an important personal goal for me, I don't think it is an appropriate mandate from an academic advisor.

To face the overt and covert resistance of medical culture, women medical students from both the last century and this one have banded together in friendships. Several of the fifteen women in Reed and Sabin's class met regularly to study together, while a series of letters between Reed and Long makes it clear that they were very close friends who supported and guided each other through their careers. Indeed, as Shrager observes, the Reed-Long relationship developed along mentor-protégé lines, with the former playing an influential role in the latter's career decisions.[23] Similarly, I, too, found that the only way I could get through the difficult process of medical school was to rely upon my small circle of female friends. However, I did not find either collegial or professional mentors of the Reed-Long variety. While there were a dearth of female professors who seemed willing to nurture female students in any meaningful way, I also did not find that women of my position were all that willing to mentor younger students. As a second-year medical student I myself was assigned a first-year "little sib" to mentor, share notes with, and otherwise support. Interestingly enough, my "little sib" was not only a woman, but an Indian American woman like me. However, our relationship barely got off the ground. After trying to set up lunches with her a few times, and being rebuffed on the grounds that she needed to study every waking moment and could not spare any time for even food, I gave up. Her shrill voice and nervous, studious manner were too much for me to bear. My "little

23 Ibid., 565.

sib" was too much of a "gunner" for me. She represented the sort of competitive student that I couldn't stand, the sort of student that made the medical school environment difficult for me. Rather than feeling like mentoring her, I wanted to run away from her. My protégé was the kind of person who made me need a mentor myself.

On the opposite end of the mentor-protégé spectrum is a good female friend from childhood who is now a surgical resident. She recently told me a story about a woman medical student on her team who had neglected pre-rounding with her on a particularly complicated patient and thus forgot to mention many relevant problems during attending rounds. My friend, because of this student's negligence, was chewed out by her attending. In return, my friend told me, she "almost tore the girl a new one." The bitter reality of surviving day to day had made my hitherto warmhearted and sensitive friend the least desirable female mentor imaginable. She herself is astounded, as are, I'm sure, many women, by the transformation. "I can't believe it," she revealed to me. "I'm a bitch on wheels." Then added, "I feel bad about myself all the time—in the O.R., on the wards, as a woman, as a doctor. I am so broken down that I can hardly support myself, much less somebody else. Every time a whiny patient gets on my nerves, I just want to slap them silly." Hardly, I'm sure, a desirable response from a physician. But it goes to show how the medical environment creates selfishness. A needy patient or a needy protégé just means less energy to take care of oneself in a hostile situation.

Relationships with men, both as friends and lovers, are equally important in surviving medical training. While I was lucky enough to have a few close male friends, I also met my husband during medical training. Indeed, many different couples emerged from my medical school class, and more than ten out of 120 students married classmates. This is perhaps one arena where we modern women have had less difficulties than our historical counterparts. Neither Reed, Sabin, nor Long mentioned any friendships with men in their journals and letters. Indeed, they seemed rather socially isolated, living together in a ladies' dormitory with nurses and other female paramedical staff. This isolation was also seen in the romantic arena. Although she eventually married, Dorothy Reed wrote in her journal, "Please God I shall stay single for the rest of my days." Long and Sabin actually did remain single for the rest of their lives, at Shrager's interpretation—"because they were afraid to be diverted by a man's attention, they sacrificed all social intercourse with men." Of course, although Shrager seems to believe they were both heterosexual, there is nothing to prove that this isolation from men did not occur as a result of sexual orientation. Regardless, studying medicine in the 1890s was so antithetical to standard feminine gender roles that no matter what their actual orientation, those early female physicians' sexualities were probably called into question. This reality was evident in their conversations with each other. Reed actually advised Long to "be as womanly as you feel, and feel as womanly as you are." On the other hand, Reed wrote "of all the women I have known she [Long] had no feminine traits ... she could have been a man."[24] Clearly, gender stereotyping was not committed solely by men.

At the end of my first year of medical school, there occurred a defining incident that thereafter determined my

[24] Ibid.

understanding of gender relations in medicine. As part of Hopkins's much touted "new curriculum," the very same one which had lured me into believing that the traditional institution had suddenly become interested in the humanities, we took a once-a-week class on medical ethics and other "social" subjects. During one such class our lecturer was Dr. Rhonda Dover, a well-known communications expert from the Hopkins school of public health. Dr. Dover, whose research is in physician-patient characteristics and communication, was to present some findings from her latest study regarding gender and doctor-patient interactions.

"Women physicians," she said, her warm, personable speaking style in stark contrast to the normally dogmatic science lectures we received in that auditorium, "have been found to take more time with their patients, and thereby engender greater trust in both male and female patients than their male counterparts."

It didn't sound that odd to me, but there was a ripple of discontent flowing like a growing wave in the class. Someone came forward to give it voice. "What do you mean, more time?"

Dr. Dover looked surprised. "More time in each interview, each examination," she explained, and then added, "We also found women to exchange more nonverbal cues of support and encouragement, and to elicit more satisfaction from their patients."

A large-necked man in the front row interrupted her. "How do you know?"

"From the taped encounters in the study," she replied, her brows slightly furrowed. "The average time was significantly greater for women physicians . . ."

"Oh, that's convenient," a disembodied male voice

from the back of the room commented. A number of female voices giggled in reply.

"You can never get women to stop talking," another man's voice boomed from a hidden corner.

There were peals of laughter. Dr. Dover, suitably shaken at this reception, started to protest. "I think it's interesting that this topic is causing so much distress in the class—" she started.

But she was cut off again. "I'm not sure if I'm exactly understanding your point, *Doctor*," a man, this time in front, in an ostensibly polite tone began.

She looked relieved at the ability to face her opponent. "What is it you don't understand?" she asked, only slightly tremulously.

From my position on the side of the lecture hall, I could see that it was a classmate I was marginally friendly with: David, an articulate fellow, a Southern gentleman, and a great favorite of the single women in our class. I was only slightly nervous about what he was going to say next. Surely, he would not allow his naturally gentlemanly character to fail him.

"I'm not sure if I understand the point of this lecture." My stomach tightened. What, for that matter, was David's point? He went on. "What kind of science is this anyway?"

"Excuse me?" Dr. Dover looked as unnerved as I felt. Was this normally genteel student calling her academic legitimacy into question?

He was. "How are you proving any of this stuff, anyway?" David asked. "Or are you just making up things that you think sound right?"

The back-row rumbling grew louder. A number of snickers gave chorus to the now louder peals of feminine giggles. I squirmed in embarrassment for the lecturer.

But it was more than that. I had been trained in social sciences; my mother was a social sciences professor. Most importantly, it was clear to me that David would not have dared to be so patronizing with a male professor, or a professor discussing nongendered topics; nor would the class have dared to be so rude. I started to feel more and more isolated, as I soon discovered the true nature of my classmates.

To give Dr. Dover credit, she took it all fairly gracefully. "What do you mean?" she asked smoothly, her emotions betrayed only by the rising flush on her cheeks. "Have you ever heard of statistics? Of social science?"

But the front-row commentator was on a roll. "I think all these findings are a little fishy, and I don't know what your point in telling us all of this is."

By this time, I couldn't hold it in anymore. Neither could the handful of other students in the class who would later join me in apologizing to Dr. Dover, and even later, in upbraiding our classmates. "What the heck are you talking about, David?" I remember myself shouting out. Others joined me in their disapproval. But our voices were drowned out by the overwhelming waves of discontent, of uproar, of chaos.

Then David clinched his argument with a well-phrased barb. It was a bomb that hit its mark, and caused an enormous roar to rise up from his platoon of similarly minded classmates. It was the worst occasion of herd aggression that I had ever seen in my medical school class, and against a professor, nonetheless. It still strikes me today as the perfect example of gendered politics in medicine.

"What are you trying to tell us, Professor?" David spat out, his voice now steely with indignation, cutting in its disrespect. "Are you trying to tell all of us intelligent, educated men in this room that you want us to . . . what—" Here, he paused, and turned around from his spot up front to gesture expressively to his audience. Then, he delivered his punch line, "What do you want us to do—*become women?*"

The room exploded with laughter. I was stunned. It was so unthinkable that men could have anything to learn from female physicians' styles of interview or patient care that even statistically proven facts were dismissed with a guffaw. Dr. Dover, as I recall, didn't finish her lecture that day. She looked shaken and upset when she left the room, and it wasn't until two years later, when I was enrolled as an MPH student at the public health school, that I would ever discuss that awful lecture with her.

"Oh, I remember that day," she said when I brought up the topic. "It was like a flashback to another century."

For an instant, the image of a turn-of-the-century medical school painting came into my mind. It's an artist's rendition of a medical lecture, and it depicts grim-faced, black-coated physicians all huddled around the figure of a half-dressed female patient who falls back into one of their arms in an apparent faint. Her eyes are closed, her breast exposed—she is the passive palate of feminine biology for them to dissect, categorize, and understand. She is certainly not their teacher, nor does she convey any information that is contrary to their already fixed beliefs about her.

If, I wonder, that hapless, gauzy-haired, bare-bosomed woman were to arise from her slumber and join the ranks of the physicians-in-training, or worse still, trade places with their illustrious teacher, would the figures in that painting push her off the canvas? Or would they allow her to stay, with the understanding that she would try her hardest to become like them, and that there would be another fainting wretch in her place who she would in turn scrutinize?

At the end of the twentieth century, women in medicine aren't willing to play any more by rules that weren't created by, or for, us. While I acknowledge the debt we have to our foremothers, I cannot, like Dorothy Reed, so easily conclude that, during our medical education, we as women "were tolerated and on the whole treated well."[25] Nor do I think it necessary to essentialize the "nurturing" qualities of some monolithic femininity and re-create an artificial "feminine medicine." Rather than looking backward, to women who were female physicians, or those who were proponents of a "feminine medicine," it is time to look forward to a humanitarian medicine, which incorporates the cultures, styles, agendas, and priorities of all of its members; a medicine not re-creating the politics of centuries past, but reinventing itself for a new millennium.

[25] Ibid., 567.

Conclusion

In 1873, Professor Edward H. Clarke, Professor of Materia Medica at Harvard Medical School, concluded that higher education for women leads to "[M]onstrous brains and puny bodies; abnormally active cerebration and abnormally weak digestion; flowing thoughts and constipated bowels."[26] Regardless of the fact that medical school may still tend to upset the digestive tracts of its male and female students, medical attitudes to women have obviously changed since Dr. Clarke's time. Although sexist jokes and comments can still be heard around the hospital corridors, it is clear that modern medical sexism manifests itself in less obvious ways. However, despite the fact that the gender war has moved away from hand-to-hand combat and adopted more sophisticated, stealth bomb–like techniques, it is critical that those of us within the medical profession work to recognize and dismantle the subtle culture of medical sexism. For those of us who are not health care providers,

[26] E. H. Clarke, *Sex in Education or A Fair Chance for the Girls* (Boston, Mass.: Osgood, 1873), as quoted in Carola Eisenberg, "Women Doctors: Where do we come from? What are we? Where are we going?" *Annals of Behavioral Science and Medical Education* 3, no. 1 (Spring 1996): 7–13.

but clients of the health care system, it is important to be well informed and vigilant. The same culture that undermines female physicians and trainees creates an environment unhealthy to patients. By dismantling medical militarism, we not only make medical training kinder and gentler for female recruits, but we change aggressive language, behavior, and customs, which too often pit the physician soldier against the patient enemy.

In writing this collection of essays, I have come to recognize and name the oppressive forces around me: the physician teacher who does not call on female students, the medical team that makes fun of its more disadvantaged patients, the mentors who should be, yet are not, there. Luckily, I have also been able to notice the perhaps hidden sources of support within the medical establishment: sensitive doctors, the nonphysician staff, and even the patients themselves. In recognizing the problem, I have also been given a glimpse of the solution.

"The experience of writing about medical school while going through it has changed my medical education tremendously," writes Perri Klass. "I have found that in order to write about my training so that people outside the medical profession can understand what I am talking about I have had to preserve a certain level of naiveté."[27] In writing *Her Own Medicine*, I have had a similar experience to Dr. Klass's. In addition, I have found that in preserving my naiveté, I have also rediscovered my sense of humor. While the gender inequities and militaristic culture of medicine initially provoked in me a sense of horrific outrage, in examining my medical school experiences more closely, I have been able to see

---

[27] Klass, *A Not Entirely Benign Procedure*, 16.

the humor in the oftentimes ridiculous antics that medical professionals and trainees accept as normal. In keeping some degree of emotional and psychological distance, I have been given a delicious vantage point to the world of medicine from which to observe and scribble.

The lesson, for me, is to retain some piece of that naiveté that allows me to see problems in what others consider normal. I have also, however, gained some degree of perspective from experience. I know now that change in medical education may not come with the breakneck speed of a revolution. However, a slow but steady changing of the guard is occurring. The weapons of this new revolution are observation, communication, and perhaps, ultimately, humor. The Emperor is powerful, but even he will turn and run at the people's ridicule. By removing layers of tradition, military culture, and anti-woman sentiment from the medical profession, we can perhaps strip away the Emperor's old clothes, and make way for a new, more egalitarian, cultural garb. We can render the Emperor, if not dead, at least obsolete. Long live the Empress. Long live her own medicine.

*If you enjoyed an inside look at
the life of a young doctor, you won't
want to miss . . .*

INTENSIVE CARE
The Story of a Nurse

As a veteran of coronary care and emergency room nursing, author Echo Heron provides a compelling insider's look into the workings of a hospital. Here is one nurse's true story, filled with all the tragedy, drama, and triumph experienced in a life dedicated to healing.

by Echo Heron

Published by The Ballantine Publishing Group.
Available at a bookstore near you.

CONDITION CRITICAL
The Story of a Nurse Continues

Echo Heron continues her engrossing chronicle of the high-pressured life of a nurse. The convict who must recover in time for his own execution and the young woman, paralyzed in a tragic accident, who vows to walk out of the hospital are just two of the remarkable people you will meet in these pages. This unforgettable account of medicine from the trenches will stay with you long after the last page has been turned.

by Echo Heron

Published by The Ballantine Publishing Group.
Available at your local bookstore.